BRAVE, BEAUTIFUL AND BARING IT ALL

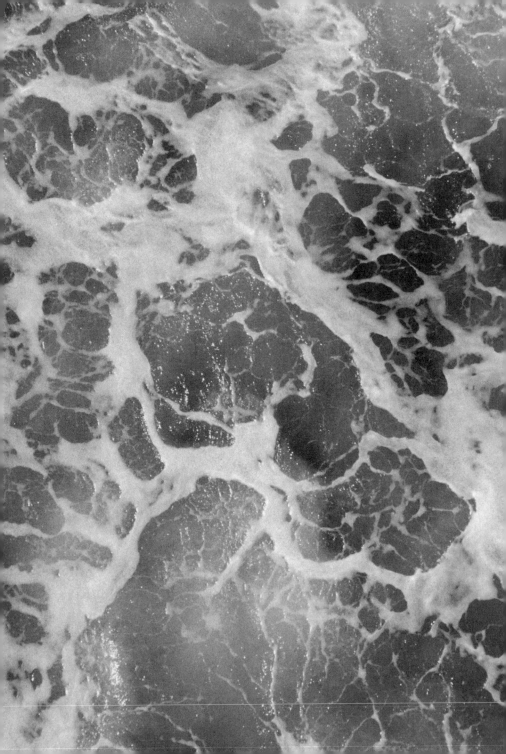

BRAVE, BEAUTIFUL

Opening Our Hearts to Happiness
No Matter What Life Throws At Us

AND BARING IT ALL

Rhyanna Watson

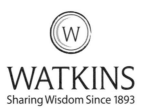

WATKINS
Sharing Wisdom Since 1893

This edition first published in the UK and USA in 2020 by
Watkins, an imprint of Watkins Media Limited
Unit 11, Shepperton House
89-93 Shepperton Road
London N1 3DF

enquiries@watkinspublishing.com

1 3 5 7 9 10 8 6 4 2

Interior designed by Francesca Corsini
Typsetting by Karen Smith
Printed and bound in the UK by TJ International Ltd.

A CIP record for this book is available from the British Library
ISBN: 978-1-786782-89-2

www.watkinspublishing.com

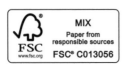

TO THE MAGICAL WORLD IN WHICH WE LIVE AND TO MY AWESOME DAUGHTER, LAINE — MY HEART-BEATER, LIGHT-GIVER, REASON WHY AND MIRACLE.

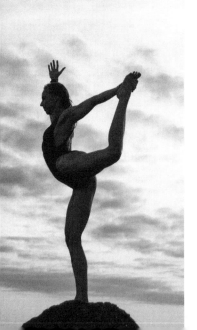

CONTENTS

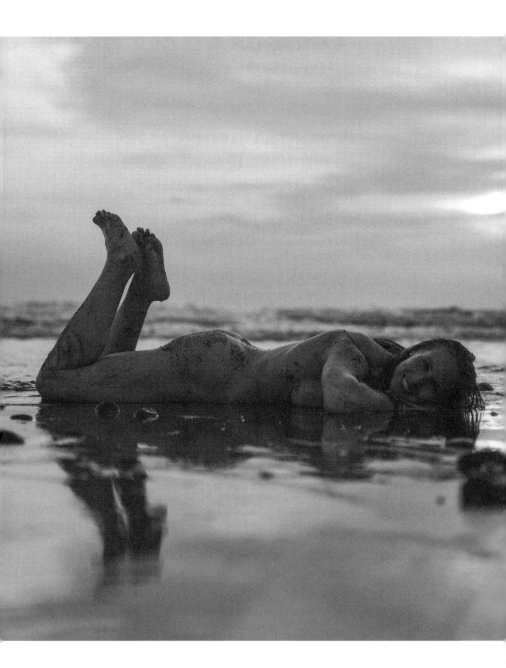

HELLO AND WELCOME!

I'd like to start by thanking you for being here, you beautiful human – and by reminding you that You Are Awesome! Life is one hell of a ride. It can be tough, sad, unfair, chaotic and confusing at times, but it's also breathtakingly beautiful and worth it.

If you don't already know me from my Open Hearts Can Unite web pages, I'm Rhyanna. I'm a mum, yoga teacher, fitness trainer, wellness consultant, Instagrammer, YouTuber and a person who – like most of us – has experienced pain and heartbreak, as well as incredible joy and love. Essentially, I'm just a woman who's trying to do her best, and I'd like to share with you some of the discoveries I've made along the way in the hope that they might help you experience more love, lightness and freedom when you most need them; feel better on a bad day, even if only a little; and accept and embrace yourself just as you are, in the knowledge that you're beautiful and you're enough.

I started my Instagram page and YouTube channel – Open Hearts Can Unite – in 2014 with the intention of having a space to express myself from the heart in a world where that can often feel tough to do – including showing images of my own body to encourage others to accept theirs. I had worked in the world of fitness training for several years by this stage, so it felt like a natural extension to share some of the experience I had gained online. Plus I had started exploring yoga just the year before and was feeling inspired by the incredible soulful way in which it was allowing me to reconnect with my body, mind and heart after an extended period of trauma, disconnection, sadness, darkness and depression that had led to an attempt on my own life.

Little did I know what an impact sharing my thoughts, images, movements and mind-body experiences online would end up having on my life. I have been blown away by the following that my pages have attracted, and I'm immensely grateful for the incredible engagement and daily interaction that I now have.

Having gone through tough times, including physical and mental abuse, sexual assault, a miscarriage, post-natal depression and the fallout from my suicide attempt, I could simply never have imagined myself ending up online helping *other* people. Yet that's where I find myself now – feeling stronger and more vibrant than ever before since coming to the simple but life-changing realization that fitness and happiness come not from our belongings, our dress size or any other external factors – but from the inside out.

To be honest, after having my beautiful daughter Laine in 2013, I struggled so much physically, as well as emotionally, that I never thought I'd have the confidence to wear a bikini again even in the privacy of my own backyard, never mind be happy to share so much of myself in online fitness content. But I have come to realize through a lot of honest soul-searching – aided by the regular practice of gorgeous yoga and dance – that this was just one of many limiting beliefs that I had subconsciously taken on from the media and other societal input. Now more than ever I realize that life's too short to be held back by such beliefs and not to feel good within yourself – as we will only ever be as beautiful as we feel. I therefore decided to cast such self-limiting beliefs to the side, get brave and get real – both about my thoughts and emotions, *and* about my body, rather than constantly hiding part of myself away! And once I started sharing my "naked truth" from this open, honest, and sometimes sensual place – driven by love and gratitude for my body, rather than fear and shame about it – my message started to resonate with a lot of others who were also in search of more raw authenticity. And so an online community of like-minded souls started to emerge.

But believe me, the journey hasn't always been easy, as presenting myself so openly and honestly – from all different angles; in all states of dress *and* undress; sometimes tired, sometimes energized; sometimes goofy, sometimes sexy; sometimes serious, sometimes playful; sometimes in a bikini, sometimes naked – has also made me vulnerable to a lot of judgement, misconception, hostility, sexual commentary and abuse, as I will share throughout the book.

To be honest, the level of trolling has been so hurtful at times that I am often asked why I continue – and why I bother to address people who don't understand what I do. I have thought a lot about this, and I guess the answer is that I know I would be doing myself and others, including my daughter and the rest of her generation, a deep injustice if I didn't continue to use my voice to try to make a difference about something that I view as so important: our capacity to live a life of love and joy in which we are accepted and respected for whoever and whatever we are, instead of one of fear and hatred in which we are judged and shamed.

SO WHO AM I?

I was born in Hobart, Tasmania. I've always loved health and fitness – I started walking at nine months and never stopped moving from there! As a teenager, I played water polo and swam for Tasmania, and competed in track events at the 2000 Pan-Pacific Games. After school, I became an executive assistant in the corporate world, which it took me a while to realize wasn't for me! Then, in 2008, I gained a personal training qualification, which gave me the chance to work with private clients before becoming fitness director on a cruise ship.

In 2012, I suffered a miscarriage, which left me feeling sad and numb. Then, in 2013, I had a beautiful baby girl – gorgeous Laine (pronounced Lay-Nee) – but I felt lost, disconnected and overwhelmed with what I now know was post-natal depression. That same year, we moved to Saudi Arabia for my partner's work and a new experience. It was hard being so far from home while I tried to figure out this new thing called motherhood. The depression got worse and I spiralled into a place of despair that ultimately led to an attempt on my own life in 2014. While this period was immensely painful to go through, it was, ironically, only at this lowest point that I was able to realize I had been living in a way that simply didn't feel true to myself. It was therefore at this time that I started to look *inside* myself for answers and rebuild a new life based on this. It was also during this time that I discovered yoga, which I genuinely believe saved my soul and which I have practised regularly ever since. It took me until 2018 before I did my yoga teacher training – with Blissology. And this has now allowed me to offer both general fitness *and* yoga programmes online. I feel deeply grateful not only to get to practise my love of movement in my daily life but also to use it to help other people feel better in *their* lives by doing this.

On the page opposite you'll see what I like to call my "My Naked Truth Statement". I created this based on everything I've just shared with you and more, to help me accept and love who I am at the core. A little later on (see pages 58–9), I will be encouraging you to create your own version of this to help *you* fully accept and love yourself too – and therefore live your best, most contented life.

My Naked Truth Statement

I'm Rhy

I'm a yoga teacher and wellbeing consultant

I taught myself pole dancing

I have experienced abuse, been raped and
tried to commit suicide

I lost a baby

I have a beautiful daughter

I post regular photos and videos of myself online,
with commentaries on life, love and yoga

I view my body as a gift and don't feel that
clothes should define us

My images, with or without clothes,
are about art and freedom

My heart hurts from all the judgement in the world

I wish I could fix it so my daughter
didn't have to experience this hatred

It's hard being misunderstood in my yoga and fitness

The judgement can be overwhelming but all I can do
is show my journey and let others share theirs

I used to be terrified of being my true self -
honest and vulnerable

But I'd rather be judged for my truth than for
something "perfect" that's not who I really am

And this is just part of my story…

WHY DID I WRITE THIS BOOK AND HOW MIGHT IT HELP YOU?

If you follow me online, you'll know I want everyone to discover how enjoying movement and being comfortable in both your body and mind aren't unattainable or unrealistic goals, irrespective of your physical fitness. Everyone deserves to feel at home in themselves.

THE DECISION TO WRITE

When people first started to suggest that I write a book with this in mind, I wasn't sure, especially given the mixed reactions that my online profile can attract. But the more I thought about it, the more I could see the potential value in sharing the lessons I've learned from my own experiences in a book rather than only in online snippets. It would give me a chance to put everything in one easy-to-view place and hopefully reach more people in a different way. So I decided to get out of my own way, drop my insecurities and go for it!

As I hope the title – *Brave, Beautiful and Baring It All* – suggests, I would love for you to go through life feeling both as brave and as beautiful as possible, knowing that there's no need to be afraid of "baring it all", by which I mean simply finding the strength to be the most authentic version of yourself, whatever others may think.

A JOURNEY OF SELF-DISCOVERY

Although the visual element of my online posts often tends to become the focus of attention due to how people view me in the poses and movements – whether super-strong, flexible, provocative or whatever other labels people choose to give me – neither my web pages nor this book are a guide to achieving the perfect *asana* (yoga pose) or a handbook for physical fitness and flexibility; and neither are they a guru's guide to happiness and enlightenment. You'll find no rules, prescriptions or expert, enlightened teachings.

Instead, I'm keen for my posts and the chapters in this book to act like stepping stones, inviting you on a journey of self-discovery – helping you get to know yourself better and love yourself more. Taking you out of your head and more into your body and heart. Helping you feel more brave and beautiful every day. Encouraging you to be bold enough to "bare it all" – guiding you to whatever it is that makes *you* feel more open, vibrant, contented and free.

FINDING YOUR TRUTH

My hope is to provide you with the space to go on a journey towards your own unique truth. This might take you to some challenging places along the way, as it has done for me. But, as I've discovered on my own journey, it's far better to be judged for your own truth and passion than for something you're *trying* to be because it's what you feel you *should* be. I have come to realize that there is great strength and courage in honesty, openness and vulnerability. I wish we could all be a lot less afraid – and more welcoming – of these qualities in life.

OPENING YOUR HEART

A fulfilling life requires us to get in the rowboat and pick up the oars, rather than just seeing where the tide takes us. My hope is that this book encourages at least one person today to recognize their ability to pick up the oars and start rowing – knowing they can go anywhere they want and be anything they choose. The power to create happy lives for ourselves, full of love, joy and connection, lies in our own hands and hearts once we get ourselves what I like to call "fit from the inside out"...

FITNESS FROM THE INSIDE OUT: BODY, MIND, HEART AND SOUL

Fitness has always been an integral part of my life. For years I thought I was as fit and strong as could be, having trained as an athlete throughout my teenage years and competed at a national level in water polo, swimming and also track events for the state of Tasmania.

CHANGING OUR ATTITUDES

Looking back, I took immense pride in my level of physical fitness and how it allowed my body to look. But as I got older and started to experience more of life's inevitable challenges – and particularly after my depression and resulting suicide attempt in 2014 – I began to realize that fitness is by no means only about physical exercise and keeping your body in good shape. Instead, fitness begins on the inside, with our minds, hearts and souls, as it's here that we need to build optimal strength, stamina, flexibility and resilience in order to sustain a happy body, whatever that may look and feel like for you, and deal with everything that life throws at us.

LOOKING INWARDS

Thinking about it now, "Fitness from the inside out" could work as an alternative title for this book, as it's essentially what I'd like to encourage you to develop for yourself, rather than focusing on the external, tangible aspects of life as many people tend to do these days, particularly when engaging with the likes of social media.

Creating fitness from the inside out means looking inwards, exploring what we're really about at the core, and learning to choose the beliefs, behaviours and actions that best serve this. It means letting go of past and current societal conditioning – beliefs we have inherited from around us that might be holding us back – and instead choosing to believe in, show up for and invest in our *own* dreams, once we've figured out what they are, of course! We can't change the world around us without first winning any wars taking place inside.

DEDICATING YOURSELF TO YOU

One of the keys to getting fit – whether on a physical, mental, emotional or spiritual level – is self-discipline. While self-discipline can feel like a difficult concept to many, really it's just about self-love, which is central to bringing about any meaningful change and a sense of achievement in your own life. It involves shifting your focus to do whatever it is that makes your heart come alive, and making the compassionate choice to dedicate yourself, your time and your energy to you and your innermost dreams.

When we commit to ourselves, we commit to any change we want. It was only when I hit rock bottom that I realized nobody could save me except me – so I'd better start investing in myself! Only then did I find yoga, teaching myself at home on my mat amidst the chaos of motherhood and daily life. It took five years of discipline and hard work to get where I am today, but, boy, was it worth it. My yoga practice – and the sense of focus and purpose it gave me – ended up turning my life around, and it still excites me every day.

WHY YOGA?

Many people who follow me online ask me why I practise and teach yoga as part of my fitness programmes. It's important to realize that, although the sometimes impressive-looking physical poses are the visible element of a yoga practice, it's not about the poses alone. For me, the focus is more on the flow of the breath, which acts as a tool to calm the thoughts and bring the mind – and therefore body and soul – back into balance. The word yoga actually means "union", hinting at its underlying aim of bringing about a sense of harmony across mind, body, heart *and* soul.

THE POWER OF BREATH AND MOVEMENT

As I mentioned earlier, I feel that yoga literally saved my life when I started practising it as part of my recovery after the attempt on my own life. Being so far away from family with a new baby was tough – especially in a culture that felt not only so different from home, but that was also very restricting for Western women. So I decided to channel my pain into a goal of developing better strength and flexibility. To achieve this, I signed up to an online yoga course to learn handstands. This started out as a purely physical thing, but soon became so much more as I experienced the breath and movement connecting my body, mind, heart and soul, creating a deeply healing and transformative practice in which I felt everything was okay again.

RECONNECTING WITH OURSELVES

This sense of feeling at one with myself was incredible. I started experiencing my senses again after years of having felt numbed by the trauma and pain of past abuses. It was as if the flow of the breath and movement had woken me from a dream, or rather a nightmare. I started to see, accept and love myself again, and the *physicality* of the practice, combined with the sense of internal calm and space it gave me, encouraged me to start embracing my full sensuality as a woman rather than hiding from this and trying to fit into society's often one-dimensional definition of how female beauty is "meant to be".

Now, here I am, a few years later, doing more than I ever dreamed and feeling happier than ever before. So I'd like to share this gift with you – so that, together, we can continue to learn, grow and thrive.

RECOGNIZING THE MIRACLE INSIDE

A big part of being fit from the inside out is simply realizing that everything you've ever needed has always been inside of you. You don't have to change, achieve or create anything. You just have to say "yes" and open yourself up to the gift within. Yet it can be so hard to say yes to ourselves. This is when we need to find the self-discipline to love ourselves – to show up, stay the course, and overcome the obstacles that we may have inherited in our thinking. So I hope that some of the messages I share within the pages that follow will encourage you even in some small way with this.

AWAKENING OUR BODIES

Fitness from the inside out can lead to an incredible new relationship with our bodies; I know it did for me. As I felt my mind–body connection strengthen with my new regular yoga practice, I felt a gradual but life-changing shift from thinking (and feeling conscious) *about* my body to thinking (and feeling in tune) *with* my body. And this shift felt not only beautiful but immensely liberating.

Once I felt at ease in myself in this way – able to feel into and love every part of myself – I began to rebuild a connection to the core of who I am and feel an urge to move through life with more gratitude and sensuality; less worry and shame. And by not caring what others thought or said, and choosing to celebrate my body both in real life and on my web pages, I could feel myself start to live with my soul as my guide, my truth as my compass.

For me, there are certain times in my daily practice when my body no longer feels separate from my mind and soul, but part of a greater, overarching oneness. And this profound experience can begin with the simplest step: becoming more aware of your breath.

"BELIEVE IN THE MIRACLE INSIDE"

OUR BREATH IS OUR LIFE: WE ARE ALL YOGIS

Whether we realize it or not, we all practise yoga every day through the simple act of breathing. With each inhale and exhale, we are engaging with what is known in yogic terms as *prana*, or our life force – viewed as not only the energy of who we are but the primal force of all creation. With each breath we take, we could therefore choose to view ourselves as yogis, taking part in the power of all creation.

BECOMING AWARE OF OUR BREATH

It was only when I started yoga at 31, after my suicide attempt, that I realized the immense power of the breath. My daughter, Laine, was two years old and I felt like a failure as a mother, that nobody loved me as a human, and that I'd be better off gone. Thankfully, I failed in the attempt to take my own life and end my own breath. And this failure marked the start of my journey with yoga and my deeper appreciation of the incredible art of breathing, which we all have the privilege of participating in every day yet rarely take the time to even notice.

As I developed a more regular yoga practice and got used to being more aware of my breath, and working with it, I soon realized that I could use these same breath-awareness techniques both to help control my panic attacks and also to help get me out of my overthinking head, back into connection with the immediacy of my body when depression was starting to take me over again.

Through slowing down and connecting with my breath, I realized that everything was okay: it was okay not to be perfect; there was no need to feel bad or be ashamed about anything; it was better to be here for Laine than not!

BEING AN OBSERVER

The art of conscious breathing is simply to observe the breath in each moment, watching the air as it enters and leaves the body. The word "observe" is key here, as it means simply watching, being aware of and accepting, rather than judging anything as good or bad.

Everything is neutral. Nothing needs a label. In this way, yoga becomes a moving meditation.

EMBRACING THE HERE AND NOW

Breath work soothes my mind, body and soul. Creating the physical asanas with the breath each day reminds me that limits can always be overcome despite what our heads might try to tell us. As I like to remind myself at times: the word "impossible" really stands for "I'm possible"!

And the great thing is that you don't have to get on a mat to reap the benefits of this side of yoga. You can begin wherever you are simply by taking time to tune into the breath and the present moment – whether you are in an asana, walking the dog or doing the washing-up. Just bring your awareness to what you are doing, breathe into your body and your actions, and remind yourself that the incredible air we breathe cradles our precious planet, gives us life and connects us with every other human being.

LETTING GO

With each inhale, take in all that is, and with each exhale, let go of all that no longer serves you, whether physical, mental or emotional.

With regular practice, this will allow the voice of your inner chatter to quieten down, leaving a sense of peace and stillness where you will be able to start to uncover your own truths and wisdoms – the ultimate key to mental and emotional freedom once you find the strength and courage to live by them.

OUR BODY AS A SANCTUARY

For me, the deepest value in the art of conscious breathing lies in the fact that it returns me to my body and allows me to feel deeper into my being so that I feel truly blessed and "at home" in myself again. I hope that you, too, get to experience the beauty of this feeling of your body as your sanctuary despite all else that may be going on in life.

As I breathe my way through the flow of my daily fitness routine, I can put all my worries aside and just be me – the perfectly imperfect human that I am – wearing whatever I'm wearing (or not) at that particular time, and trying my best to follow my heart, support others, and promote more beauty and unity in the world.

JUST BEING YOURSELF

For example, while it can sometimes hurt more than I can say to be misjudged and hated on the way I often am for how I present myself online – or rather for how others choose to *view* what I present as sexually provocative rather than natural and sensual – I try to breathe through it all with love and compassion, in the knowledge that my decision since my suicide attempt to just be myself, in all my glory – mess or goddess, with clothes or without, liked or not liked... – is what makes me feel brave, beautiful, alive and worthwhile.

And the right for everyone to simply be *themselves* – whatever that might be – without fear of judgement or shaming is ultimately what I stand for. So if ever you find it tough to just be yourself due to external expectations and pressures, you may well find it useful to start exploring the art of "Watching the breath" (see overleaf).

It's my hope that regular practice of this simple exercise could start to shift things for you in the same amazing way as it did for me, so you, too, can start to sit in your own authenticity with the ease and confidence that each and every one of us deserve.

WATCHING THE BREATH

It's always worth taking a few moments to bring your conscious attention to the breath that sustains you when you can – to help you feel calmer, more present in the moment and more connected to your body. A bonus is that you can do this anywhere – on the way to work, on a park bench, when you wake in the morning, while cooking a meal... Here are a few simple steps to get you started:

1. Find a quiet space where you won't be disturbed for a few minutes. Give yourself permission to dedicate this time to you. Turn off your phone and switch off any screens.

2. Sit comfortably, with your hands placed gently on your lap, palms facing up.

3. Relax your gaze so that you are not focusing on anything in particular. If you prefer, close your eyes.

4. Tune into your breathing. Don't try to change it. Just become aware of the air entering and leaving your body through your parted lips and your nostrils.

5. As you relax into this, become aware of the rise and fall in your body with each inhale and each exhale. Become aware of what is happening in your whole being.

6. Gradually let your breathing settle until it feels relaxed, quiet and fairly deep.

7. Simply let thoughts come and go, like watching butterflies on the breeze or waves on the shore.

8. If you find your mind wandering, gently bring it back to your breath. Silently tell yourself: "Now I am breathing in. Now I am breathing out."

9. Observe everything as if in slow motion. Breathe in this rare air. You feel alive. You are yourself. You are truly, finally, always yourself. And that's enough.

10. When you are ready, steady your gaze and allow yourself to return to everyday life, knowing that this sense of calm is waiting for you any time you need it.

Note that, near the end of the book, on pages 148–153, you'll also find a range of seven simple breathing meditations based on the exercise above, each one focusing on the theme of one of the seven chapters.

DEVELOPING BODY POSITIVITY

Another important topic I want to address as part of getting fit from the inside out is that of body positivity: a wonderful growing social movement that challenges the ways in which society presents and views the physical body, based on the belief that everyone deserves to have a positive body image and feel good about themselves.

CHALLENGING STEREOTYPES

In Western culture, stereotypes of the "perfect" tall, slim, toned body tend to dominate mainstream media. And anything that doesn't conform to these unrealistic visions of "perfection" are often treated, whether consciously or not, as sub-standard. Thankfully, things are starting to change, what with the rise of the body positivity movement, but unfortunately we still have a long way to go – especially women, about whom we see daily body-shaming headlines, whether around size, shape, cellulite, or whatever other physical attributes the media feel they have the right to comment on and criticize that day.

IT'S ALL IN OUR PERCEPTION

To anyone out there who feels worried, self-conscious or ashamed about any aspect of yourself, from your size, shape, height, skin, stretch marks, freckles, birth marks, wrinkles, pimples, hair, balding, or any other trait often associated with being "less than perfect", I feel for you. I have had many such concerns too – from feeling too muscly and "masculine" to feeling deeply unattractive during my first pregnancy due to my size and all the changes. But now is the time for us to reassess why we allow ourselves to feel this way when all we're doing is comparing ourselves against unrealistic ideals and images that have been fed to us by the media. Why are we buying into these false, and frankly harmful, perceptions that some bodies deserve more praise than others and that our differences are somehow flaws?!

Isn't it time to realize that, while we might not be able to alter certain aspects of the body we have, we *do* have the power to change our own perceptions of and feelings about them – in order to just accept and love ourselves the way we are?

ALL BODIES ARE EQUAL

If we can start to shift the conversation away from what we think is "wrong" in ourselves to what is "right" in us and what is wrong in the way society *treats* us, we may just encourage people to start celebrating *every* body as equal – no matter what size, shape, age, ethnicity or physical ability. This involves putting an end to judging, either internally or externally, both our own bodies and other people's. It means avoiding not just negative commentary and derogatory labels but also avoiding putting certain body types on a pedestal. All bodies are good bodies. All bodies are positive.

THE CHALLENGE OF BEING BODY POSITIVE

That said, becoming body positive isn't easy. Finding unadulterated self-love every day is tough when we're surrounded by pressures that continually demand we transform and conform. So, throughout this book I invite you to keep coming back to these key themes that we've explored in the introduction:
✶ getting fit from the inside out
✶ watching the breath
✶ developing body positivity
... to check in on how you feel you're doing with them and whether they are helping you feel both more brave and more beautiful each day.

YOUR JOURNEY THROUGH THIS BOOK

I hope the insights that I've provided so far give you a good idea of where I'm coming from with this book. The main chapters that follow will continue to explore similar core topics from different perspectives and in more depth in the hope that you might find some words of reassurance, guidance or even inspiration from time to time.

CHAPTERS AS STEPPING STONES

I've grouped my musings – a mixture of thoughts that I've shared online in the past and a lot of new material – into chapters (and chapter sub-sections) that I hope will be useful stepping stones on your journey of self-exploration. Each one covers traits that I see as fundamental when it comes to living life as authentically, as bravely and as beautifully as we can – treating both ourselves and others with the love and respect we all deserve in order to unite, thrive and be happy:

✱ *Laying our authentic selves bare invites us to explore how we present ourselves to the world, strip away our self-imposed restrictions, uncover our beautiful multi-faceted layers and be honest about who we really are*

✱ *Seeing the perfection in imperfection reminds us that it's okay not to be okay, the importance of love, and the risk of putting people on pedestals*

✱ *Choosing compassion over stories in our head encourages us to unravel some of the tales we tell ourselves about who we are, quieten our inner critic, and replace expectations and judgements with kindness*

✱ *Freeing our inner child helps us to welcome more curiosity and joy back into our lives, and reminds us of the power of vulnerability*

✱ *Realizing darkness allows our light to shine* helps us to accept that life can be difficult but that there are ways to meet the challenges with grace

✱ *Embracing our innate sensuality* reminds us of the difference between sensuality and sexuality, and urges us to reclaim our own bodies and sensuality, both the masculine and feminine energies

✱ *Opening our heart and loving life* brings everything together to set us even more firmly on the path to a life of love, beauty, courage and unity where both strength and vulnerability are recognized in all their glory

CREATING YOUR OWN PATH

Feel free either to read the whole book in order or to dip in at your leisure if there's a particular theme that sounds or feels relevant for a particular time. The chapters can be read in any order you like.

Throughout the book, you will find a number of practical exercises to help you more directly experience some of the concepts explored. You'll also find a scattering of motivational sayings that I hope will help to reinforce some of the key messages in the book.

TAKING THE FIRST STEPS

We can spend a lot of our lives trying to follow the same path, subconsciously programmed to believe that happiness lies in obeying rules and being like everyone else. But the good news is that there are no rules! Happiness, bravery and beauty all simply involve making a decision to live as your inner voice tells you to, irrespective of how others may view that. If you feel unhappy, with a need to apologize or explain who you are, it means the voice in your head is telling you the wrong story and it's time to get busy rewriting. My hope is that this book will help you to become the narrator of your own brave and beautiful life, willing to "bare it all" in your own unique, authentic way.

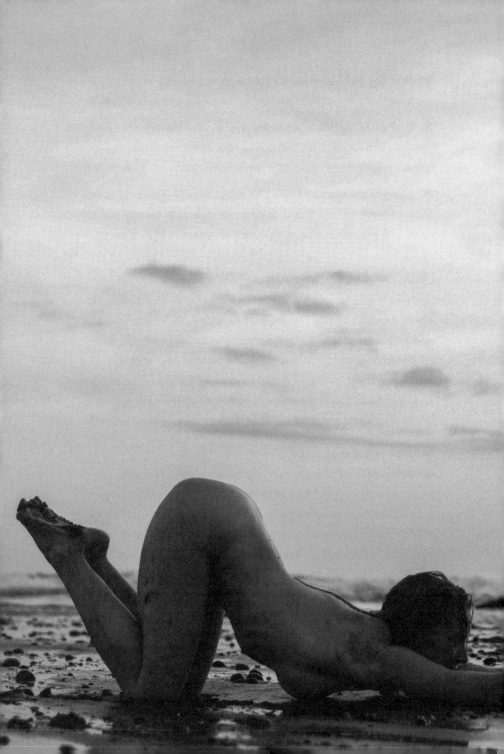

LAYING OUR AU-THENTIC SELVES BARE

CHAPTER 1:
LAYING OUR AUTHENTIC SELVES BARE

When I was a young girl I wanted to be the first female prime minister of Australia, because I wanted to change lives. Then I realized my heart and soul didn't fit this kind of job, or label. Although my passion lies in helping others, that doesn't always have to be done in the "biggest", most obvious ways. Laying our authentic selves bare means being brave enough to be honest about both our strengths and the areas in which we are perhaps not so strong; it means being ready to walk our own path in order to make our own unique contribution in the world.

Maybe if society didn't make us feel ashamed of our weaknesses and the adversities we encounter, or teach us to hide our light away; maybe if we were taught that we are being brave for sharing our true selves, that this is the most honest and human thing we could do; then maybe we would all be better at understanding ourselves and each other, and more compassionate as a whole.

In order to help us acknowledge, accept and honour who we really are underneath all the labels that the world often places on us, we will cover three main topics in this chapter:

✳ EXPLORING HOW WE PRESENT OURSELVES IN THE WORLD – are we being true to ourselves in a world obsessed with images of youth, beauty and "perfection", or are we distracted by the pressures of social media and all else?

✳ STRIPPING AWAY SELF-IMPOSED RESTRICTIONS – what would life look like if we could free ourselves from our own limited self-perceptions, and dare to own our hidden power?

✳ UNCOVERING OUR MUTLI-FACETED LAYERS – how much better would we feel if we could accept that we are complex beings, full of contradictions, rather than trying to fit the narrow perceptions and expectations of others?

It isn't the stuff on the surface that will make us feel beautiful; it's knowing and loving ourselves. The confidence we develop as we lay our authentic selves bare – vulnerable, broken, yet real – is what will make us both look and feel beautiful from within.

EXPLORING HOW WE PRESENT OURSELVES IN THE WORLD

The notion of what we are at our core and how we choose to present this to the world is an interesting one, especially in today's culture of reality television and social media, in which boundaries between private and public personas have become so blurred, and so many people spend time connecting with strangers through screens.

LIFE ON SCREEN

Technology can create amazing opportunities to reach out, befriend, learn and grow, but it can also cause us to struggle under the pressure of unrealistic expectations and ideals that lead us to present an image of what we think *others* might want, or what might help us fit in, rather than what we really believe in ourselves. In a world that often pushes us towards robotic perfection, it can take all our bravery to even get to know our authentic selves, never mind to lay ourselves bare.

Take a moment to consider: How authentic do you feel in the way you present yourself to the world, both in real life and online? Would you still be doing the same things, saying the same things and taking the same photos if social media weren't rolling? Would you continue to chase your dreams if you were the only one who knew about them?

I ask myself the same question every day. My answer is "yes" because even before the days of social media, I was working on my fitness, strength and flexibility, getting to know my body better, exploring my sensuality, practising yoga, dancing and dreaming – just as I do now.

CHOOSING WHAT TO SHARE

It's a tricky balancing act when it comes to how much to share about ourselves on social media given the enormous reach that content can have. We are each responsible for our own online experience – and that can be challenging. Approached wisely, however, it can also be a chance to learn more about ourselves, such as how comfortable we feel merging our private and public lives. Is it important to you to differentiate between the two? Or is it better just to "be" yourself the whole time, sharing anything and everything – to avoid any sense of separation and therefore potential disconnection in your life?

ELECTRIC EGO

When it comes to how we present ourselves in the world, it's all too easy to be ruled by our ego. Do you need people to say you look good or to have a certain number of "likes" on your feeds to feel good? If you're disappointed because you only have one "like" instead of your usual 700, you only got 700 instead of your usual 1,500, or you posted something and then lost a follower, the likelihood is that you're not posting for you. This means your happiness will always be based on others, and you're letting *them* hold the power. If you relate to this, it might be a good idea to take time out and get your bearings back.

HOW DO YOU SEE *YOURSELF*?

Remember: the world won't stop if we take a break from keeping up with the Joneses. In fact, things are likely to vastly improve once we start living from our own sense of self-knowledge and authenticity again! The most important thing, after all, is being happy with how you see *yourself*. When you're confident in this, you'll have lots of scope as to how you choose to present things as you won't be affected by the number of followers you have, or what others think and say.

THE PARTS WE DON'T SEE

When I post images and videos online, I often wonder whether people consider the hard work behind them, or whether they just think of me as "the girl with the flexible body", "the girl who posts naked yoga videos" or "the Open Hearts Can Unite lady". On the whole, people tend not to contemplate everything that's likely to have led us to where we are now – in my case: a disciplined training regime, daily yoga, good nutrition and a lot of self-enquiry, on the back of much personal adversity. The simple truth is that, as authentic as we try to be, we can't understand all of a person through social media snippets!

DARING TO BARE

Sometimes I wish people could witness my behind-the-scenes struggles as a reminder that even though the yoga poses I present might look like they come easy with an athletic body like mine, I've worked hard to maintain that body. And that – although I might seem bold and brazen to some people for posting naked or semi-naked videos (and sometimes even full frontals) – sharing these posts actually still makes me feel deeply nervous and uncomfortable, which is the whole point: to push myself beyond my comfort zone.

The trick is not to shy away from such moments of discomfort or to build up barriers against them, boxing ourselves in, but to welcome the lessons they bring, working through them to strip away our self-imposed restrictions and grow beyond our limitations...

STRIPPING AWAY SELF-IMPOSED RESTRICTIONS

It often feels safe to stay in our comfort zone and play small, as there's no risk of being overcome by the power of our own greatness. Yet it's only when we start recognizing and stripping away the self-imposed restrictions in our life that we get to claim the birthright of our authentic selves and be truly happy.

IDENTIFYING OUR RESTRICTIONS

Take a little time to start considering what your most limiting beliefs and behaviours currently are, or have been in the past. At one point I felt that I was a bad mother, a useless partner, too athletic in stature ever to be thought of as feminine and beautiful, not brave enough to show people my true, damaged and vulnerable self, and not academic enough to write. Yet here I am writing a book helping people to be brave and beautiful on the back of my online profile as a wellness trainer!

KEEP BELIEVING

I truly never expected to be where I am today, teaching and engaging with such a wonderful community on Instagram and YouTube. And when I think about all the crippling beliefs that previously held me back, I realize that I had taken them on from society and internalized them to such an extent that they had started to feel like part of me!

Now, more than ever, I know that I can be whoever I want to be: I define what I am and what I can achieve – as do you, for you. So please do check in with yourself to see how you might be holding yourself back through *your* inherited conditioning. Your limitations will, of course, be completely different from mine, so just see what comes up for you.

WHAT iF?

Take a moment to think about all the things you might have achieved in the past year had you got over your various personal hang-ups, stopped expecting perfection in all areas of your life and instead just showed up at your best, at your worst, *and* at your in-between. By showing up, I mean simply letting yourself be seen for who you really are, flaws 'n' all, no holding back – fully present in the moment.

IF YOU CAN'T DO iT FOR YOURSELF...

Now that I'm a mum, my priority in life is my daughter, Laine. She pays attention to every darn thing I do. And this makes me much more self-aware than I otherwise might be. As such, I've decided that I simply don't have time for self-imposed limitations anymore, because if I do, Laine will too! And I refuse to teach her to spend her energy on toxic thoughts that she isn't good enough or on picking apart her own body. I refuse to pass that on to her. Her inner voice is counting on *my* inner voice to be strong, authentic and empowering, so that's what I'm going to make sure it is!

I often still get beaten down by my negative thoughts and self-doubts, of course, but the difference is that now I don't stay in this space for long. Instead, I stand up against them and fight – both for Laine and for me. I won't let negative, restricted thinking win.

So, if you can't do it for yourself, who is counting on you? Your mum? You best friend? Your colleagues? Your students? Believe me, there is somebody out there who needs the completely authentic you.

OVERCOMING SETBACKS

It's all too easy to slip back into self-limiting ways when we encounter setbacks of some sort. For example, as I've mentioned, when I share images of myself online, I tend to attract my fair share of criticism as well as compliments. At first when this happened, it quickly led me back to my old negative thinking patterns, wondering why anyone would ever want to listen to what I have to say in the first place. However, I soon realized that I can't possibly let my innermost worth be contingent upon either the appearance of my body or the opinions of others. I'm no longer willing to participate in conversations that contradict my authentic broader vision for my own life. I won't do it for myself. I won't do it for the sake of the person I'm talking to. Only *we* should get to define who we are, even though it's hard to stay strong at times in a world full of labels and judgements.

BEWARE OF "IF ONLYS"

Common self-judgements that I hear from clients I work with include things like "If only I was X size or Y weight, I'd be happy." But, trust me, meeting these types of external goals won't necessarily make you happy, which means that this might actually be a limiting thought cunningly disguised as a goal!

Happiness doesn't have a specific look or follow a particular exercise plan. The truth is that we have the choice to be happy right now, in this moment, whatever our size, weight and fitness level, if we're just willing to accept and love our authentic self laid bare, as we are. However, there's no reason, of course, that this should stop us from setting important health and fitness goals separately in their own right, to add to the many nuanced layers of being that make us into the beautiful, complex beings that we are...

UNCOVERING OUR MULTI-FACETED LAYERS

It may seem pretty basic, but it's important to remember that we are all a million different things rolled into one. We aren't just men, women, sisters, brothers, mothers, fathers, daughters and sons, we are also friends, colleagues, parents, lovers and so much more beyond. We have the capacity to be smart, sassy, sensual, silly, solemn and all manner of other things. Why, then, does it often feel like attempts are being made to put us in boxes that don't allow much room for manoeuvre? Please let's not allow the world to squeeze us into one-size-fits-all moulds. Instead, let's delight in the fact that we humans have the privilege of being all kinds of wonderful at once!

THE FULL SPECTRUM OF LIFE

My decision to present so much of myself online means that I share many aspects of my character on my pages – from fit, strong and flexible to fun, warm and friendly; from open, honest and vulnerable to playful, naughty and sensual. This sometimes involves me showing private bits of myself, and sometimes, just like in real life, showing "I have no idea why I'm doing this but it feels good" bits!

My goal is to show the full spectrum of my life, rather than either only the perfect, polished version of what society has often come to expect from ads and the like, or only the overtly sexy side of things as seen in other places. I'm not making a choice to be just one thing; I'm simply being a human and showing many aspects of my life on-screen as well as off. Yet I receive messages from people telling me that I'm "too much", "an inappropriate woman" and even "a bad mother" (can you imagine how hurtful that feels!) – not as a result of what I'm saying in my messages, but purely because of what I'm wearing and the camera angles of my body that I sometimes show.

EMBRACING ALL THAT WE ARE

To me, this kind of mean-spirited feedback shows how sadly restricted and conditioned many people's thinking has become, and why there's such a strong need for us to continue to embrace and celebrate our complex, multi-faceted selves without limits – in order to make a stand against the haters by loving each other even harder in return.

If we reject people's attempts to define us in narrow-minded ways and instead accept responsibility for all aspects of our authentic selves, we empower ourselves in the process. The "Connecting with Your Authentic Self" exercise overleaf will help you to do this with great self-compassion, setting you on the path to enhanced freedom and wholeness, so do feel free to try it any time it seems appropriate.

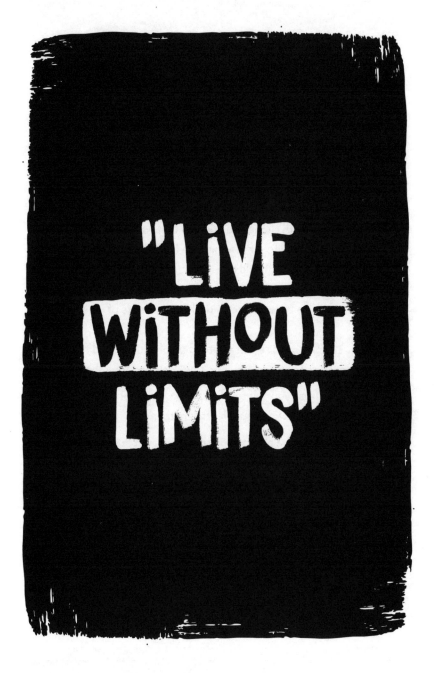

CONNECTING WITH YOUR AUTHENTIC SELF

Underneath all the conditioning that we have inherited throughout life – everything we have been told about how we "should" or could be – our contented, authentic self lies waiting to meet us. Feel free to try this exercise any time you'd like to reconnect with this deep sense of inner self.

1. Dig out a recent photograph of yourself and find a quiet space where you won't be disturbed for a short while.

2. Treat yourself to a few gentle inhales and exhales, gradually letting your breath lengthen.

3. Take the photograph that you have chosen and let your gaze rest gently on it.

4. Become aware of the sensations in your body as you look at the image – any tightening or loosening; any sudden surge of irritation or sense of soothing.

5. Continue to contemplate the image, letting any thoughts about it come and go without judgement.

6. If you find your mind wandering or any judgements creeping in, bring your attention back to your breath and the photograph.

7. Imagine a golden ball of love above your head. Take this opportunity to breathe in that love, down into your body. Send it through your touch into the image in your hands.

8. Exhale all thoughts and emotions that you feel no longer serve you as you sit here for a few moments, breathing slowly in and out.

9. Look at the person in the photograph and imagine it is a close friend. What message do you want to give to them?

10. In your thoughts, tell your friend your message, breathing in love and exhaling out all else.

11. When you are ready, steady your gaze and return to everyday life.

Our authentic selves are too beautiful and deserving to be denied, so congratulations for having made this connection!

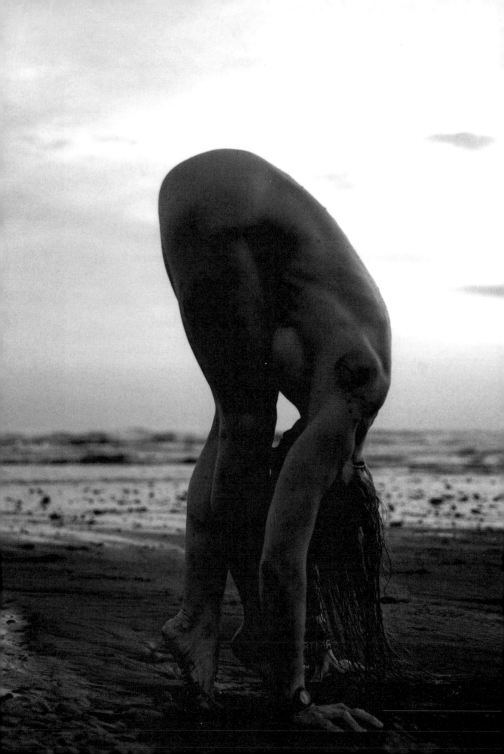

SEEING THE PER- FECTION IN IMPER- FECTION

CHAPTER 2:
SEEING THE PERFECTION IN IMPERFECTION

We are all beautiful children of the Universe – amazing just as we are, human beings sharing this incredible, diverse planet. When you consider the chances of any one of us existing here on earth, me and you together, at this time in the whole history of the entire Universe, how fantastic is that?

To be human is to be imperfectly perfect, so please let's stop comparing ourselves to friends who appear more confident, colleagues who appear more organized, or Insta-stars whose lives appear more glamorous. We all have our strengths and weaknesses. Nobody is perfect, no matter how things may look from the outside.

And, please, let's stop looking at all these photoshopped, airbrushed models in ads and wondering why we don't look like them. We're not like them because they're not representative of real women! When I look at such images, I find nothing inspiring or empowering in them because they are not genuine. They contain no flaws, no life.

But we *are* real. *You* are real. Our differences are what make us beautiful, unique and truly human. In order to encourage us all to start celebrating, rather than hiding, these unique "imperfections", we will explore three main topics in this chapter:

✳ ACCEPTING THAT IT'S OKAY NOT TO BE OKAY – why are we wasting so much time and energy trying to pretend everything is okay the whole time? Wouldn't we feel lighter if we didn't have to do this?

✳ LEARNING TO LOVE OURSELVES – how much happier would we feel if we could accept and love *all* aspects of ourselves, both our strengths and our weaknesses, and see the unique beauty in all our messy, mixed-up, individual wonderfulness?

✳ DROPPING THE NEED FOR PEDESTALS – what if we learned to celebrate all our amazing differences instead of worshipping only certain people, often only to see them fall off their pedestal when they fail to live up to our false notion of perfection?

Seeing the perfection in imperfection is about saying, "Here I am in all my glory." It involves neither running away from ourselves nor chasing an ideal: we are simply accepting and appreciating all that is. When we can begin to love and accept ourselves in this way, "flaws" 'n' all, we will open ourselves up to the infinite love of the Universe.

ACCEPTING THAT IT'S OKAY NOT TO BE OKAY

Life sure can be tough at times, with all sorts of challenges cropping up along the way, so it's understandable that we can feel "bad" at times – whether hurt, vulnerable, sad, angry, disappointed, overwhelmed or whatever else. We wouldn't be human if we didn't experience the whole range of human emotions in response to all that life throws at us.

WHY DO WE BEAT OURSELVES UP?

Some people think that it's only through experiencing the emotions at the "negative" end of the spectrum that we are truly able to appreciate the "positive" feelings, such as joy, excitement and contentment. Plus, living through experiences of negative emotions gives us a chance to work through issues and grow; many people who have gone through all sorts of tough times go on to rise up and do wonderful things. So why do we so often beat ourselves up about feeling in any way "bad" or "down"? If only we could learn to accept that it's okay not to be okay at times, we could stop spending so much energy resisting it and start dancing to the beat of our own drum.

RECOGNIZING WHEN WE'RE FALLING

That's not to say, of course, that we can't at times take action to prevent ourselves from falling into prolonged negative patterns. Destructive thoughts tend to creep up on us – notions that we are not good enough or that we need to do better.

So, it's important to remember that they are just thoughts, that's all. They are not truths. And they are just temporary, so they will pass. The next time such thoughts emerge, take a deep breath and feel your heart, your soul, your feet rooting into the world that creates your foundations for all that is. Tell yourself you are doing just fine: you are here today, living with all you have – and that is enough. Tell yourself that you are proud of you because you have always been enough.

WHERE WILL WE DEVOTE OUR ENERGY?

We can spend our lives and our energy beating ourselves up for not being this way or that way, for not having this thing or that, for not being like this person or that person, for not living up to unrealistic standards that we mistakenly think apply to all of us, or for feeling down when things don't go quite according to plan.

The thing is – as a part of all life, whether or not we know it or believe it – we are constantly giving and receiving energy. And what we give energy to grows, so if we give energy to our negative thoughts and worries – whether by wallowing in them or resisting them – they will grow. But if we instead choose to devote energy to loving and accepting ourselves, even when we're *not* feeling okay, then love and acceptance will grow and, ironically, we're likely to start feeling better.

So let's take a step back from putting ourselves down. We all struggle in some part of our lives. Here's to all of us humans doing our best, even though it doesn't always look or feel like much. No matter how it looks or feels, in the bigger picture, it's still pretty awesome.

AVOIDING COMPARISONS

Another way to prevent ourselves falling into negative slumps is to avoid the toxic trap of comparing ourselves to others, especially when we're feeling particularly vulnerable.

It's all too easy to think things along the lines of "How does she effortlessly balance work and motherhood, while I'm barely keeping it together?" and "How does he cope so well with his workload when I feel like I'm drowning with what looks like less to do?" Unhelpful

"LIVE THIS CRAZY LIFE WITH GRATITUDE FOR ALL YOU ARE"

thoughts like these feed our insecurities and, as just discussed, cause them to grow. The thing to remember, of course, is that we rarely get to see the reality behind the veneer of other people's lives, whether on- or offline. And, if we did, we might not feel so jealous or inferior, as everyone has their "stuff" to deal with and everyone feels down at times. It's just part of the fabric of life – and it's okay. It's all okay.

IT'S ALL PART OF THE JOURNEY

At some point, we will all feel dragged down in this world. We will all struggle to find our multi-faceted wholeness and accept it, imperfections and all. It can be hard to own our truth in a world that can be so quick to pass judgement on who we are – as well as who it thinks we are. This is when I tell myself to stand my ground: "It's okay to feel X and Y. It will pass. And you are going to do great things being an original; never a copy."

BEING GRATEFUL

Maybe it's time to be grateful that we have the capacity to feel so deeply, even if that does cause sadness and hurt at times. When we recognize what we *have* instead of what we *don't* have, we can celebrate ourselves for all that we are – not pull ourselves down for our bad days, our weaknesses, our flaws and who we *aren't*.

Let's look for the space between the highs and lows of life to respond calmly to the outside world, rather than react purely from our fleeting emotions. Nobody really knows our journey – or anyone else's for that matter – so let's all show one another a little more love.

LEARNING TO LOVE OURSELVES — FLAWS 'N' ALL

When you think of the words "strong", "brilliant", "awesome", "beautiful" and "loving", I want you to think of YOU. I want you to know that your love for both your self and others can and will change the world, even if you can't yet see how. If there is one thing in this world that I know for certain, it's that we are all so loved.

RECOGNIZING OUR VALUE

So now it's just a matter of believing this about ourselves, no matter what value we feel the people around us might have given us or what label social media might have placed on us.

The true measure of our value comes from our own body, mind, heart and soul feeling at home, and at ease, with who we are and what we are doing; not from what others think or project. This is what will allow us to experience true love, peace, joy and wholeness.

THE ART OF SELF-ACCEPTANCE

One way of looking at self-love is as a sincere acceptance of all that we are and have been, as well as acceptance of all that others are and have been. It is an agreement to forgive anyone who has ever hurt us, ourselves included, whether intentionally or not.

It is a pact with ourselves to make the most of the present and move on with faith that the rest of our life can be the best of our life – filled with unconditional love and compassion.

As such, learning to accept and love ourselves, flaws 'n' all, can feel like a rebirth that is more stunning than the brightest sunset.

EMBRACING OUR FLAWS

We can choose to hide ourselves because of our perceived flaws. Or we can embrace those flaws. We can choose to see how our cracks and quirks add beauty both to our lives and the world around us. And we can choose to recognize that the qualities that make us unique are something to celebrate, not suppress.

Embracing what either we or others might perceive as our "flaws" enables us to let go of any limiting beliefs, thoughts and behaviours that no longer serve us and instead make choices based on things, places and people that empower us towards more love.

STEPPING INTO OUR TRUTH

It's time to stop contorting ourselves to fit into a life that we think we should have, that others want for us or that makes us unhappy. You are a breathtakingly beautiful human and there are many people who love your magic and what you stand for.

To help you live in a more loving space on a day-to-day basis, focus on the people who make you breathe deeper, not harder – who make you feel more you, not less you, and who create space for you and your heart. And remember to do the same for them, and not to chase the people who don't give you that space and love. Life is a flow, an ebb, a losing, a finding, a disappearing, a blooming. And there is a place for us all in that, just as we are.

Home is where you are right now, and nobody can take that away from you. But only you can make the brave and beautiful decision to love you and to be you no matter what. Only you can have the courage to open your heart, allow others in and come together in the name of love, joy and happiness.

"BE WHO YOU ARE — NOT ASHAMED OF WHO YOU ARE"

CELEBRATING OURSELVES

I made a decision after attempting to take my own life to no longer fret about or fear who I am, to no longer be ashamed of my looks and to no longer feel as if I'm not enough in this world.

Instead, I made a commitment to truly loving myself, celebrating the gift of my body, mind, heart and soul, and allowing myself to simply be who I am – so that I can slowly and mindfully become the beacon of unconditional love that I believe I'm meant to be.

CELEBRATING ONE ANOTHER

I also made a conscious choice to live in the spirit of loving and celebrating all women for who they are, as we can do such immensely beautiful things when we all work together – in union, rather than in a spirit of competition, judgement and fear.

The more we can love those who are struggling and ourselves in our own struggles, the more strength we will all have to reclaim our past, heal our hearts and love our present! Let's give support back to our struggles and our scars so we can all heal. And let's see self-doubt and self-loathing for the needless, fruitless activities that they are in order to make more room for true love and acceptance of ourselves.

SHINING OUR LIGHT – SHARING OUR LOVE

Self-love is an interesting concept, as it has the word "self" in it, yet it doesn't have to be in any way a selfish thing. In fact, by loving ourselves, we will automatically have more capacity to love and uplift others. Self-love is the understanding that thousands of candles can be lit from a single flame, and the life of that flame will not be decreased either in quality or brightness. Love never decreases by being shared.

The Naked Truth Statement exercise overleaf will help you to inject your own life with a little more acceptance and self-love.

CREATING YOUR NAKED TRUTH STATEMENT

In the Introduction, I shared my Naked Truth Statement, which I wrote as a way to help me accept and love myself, flaws and all. Now I'd like to invite you to write one of your own. Here are a few tips that might help:

✱ *Your Naked Truth Statement will be personal to you – there are no rights or wrongs.*

✱ *You can write your Statement on screen, or with pen and paper, whichever you prefer.*

✱ *Be as open and honest in it as you can.*

✱ *You don't have to share it with anybody unless you want to: no one is going to judge what you write.*

✱ *Don't worry about spelling mistakes or crossing things out – just keep on writing.*

✱ *If any strong emotions surface, sit with them for a while before carrying on.*

Find a quiet moment when you won't be disturbed.
Take a few deep, calming breaths. Then, when you are
ready, start your Statement by writing your name at the
top: *I am X*. Underneath, in any order you like, write a
short sentence about each of the following and/or
anything else that you feel drawn to include:

1. What you love to do

2. What you do for a living

3. A quirky fact about you

4. An important relationship in your life

5. An important secret from your past

6. A time when you hurt a lot

7. A time when you felt really happy

8. A major fear from the past

9. A major hope for the future

These are just suggestions to get you started. Your Statement
won't define you. It can just be used to shine a little light
on the core of what makes you you and remind you what
a beautiful human you are, perfect in your imperfections.

DROPPING THE NEED FOR PEDESTALS

In our current media-driven society, there is a tendency towards putting people on pedestals, identifying them as the new picture-perfect poster boy or girl for whatever product or cause is being championed at the time. This might sound flattering at first, but unfortunately the same people who like to put us up on this pedestal often also like to knock us down. And, in some cases, they may even end up vilifying us, because that's the risk if people are viewed in all-or-nothing, black-and-white ways, rather than seeing all the many beautiful shades of grey in between.

KEEPING GROUNDED

Some of my biggest fears are about being put on a pedestal and being told by others that I am more than I am. Because I know I'm not any better than anyone else; I'm just different. I'm just myself.

I'm not here to be put on a pedestal. I'm an imperfect human, just trying to be real, connect and help others through being open, honest and sharing my experiences. More often than not, I'm the girl who's fallen off any pedestal I've been put on, and I'm sitting on the ground underneath, saying something inappropriate and turning red as a tomato while everyone laughs at my chaos!

Pedestals give me vertigo; the air can be thin up there.

THE PROBLEM WITH HERO WORSHIP

There's a whole ton of hero worship online these days – we all want to believe in something or someone. Maybe there really are some gurus out there who possess the secret to life, and if we follow them, we'll all be the wiser for it. I get it, I really do. But, all said and done, those experts are just people living life, like the rest of us. If we rely solely on them to solve any problems we have, we are giving away our power. By all means let's love them and be inspired by them, but let's keep our power where it belongs – with us.

CELEBRATING OUR DIFFERENCES

All humans are fallible, whatever their status or influence. Likewise, we all have different strengths and abilities, which is what makes us all so interesting. One person can do a better yoga backbend while another can do a better forward bend, inversion or twist. Some of us have scientific minds while others lean more towards the artistic.

Wouldn't we all be much happier if we started celebrating our many differences – and the amazing breadth and depth this brings to the world – instead of praising and worshipping some people as somehow "better" or more "worthy" than others?

RESPECTING AND ACCEPTING OUR IMPERFECTIONS

Once I decided to respect who I was with all my imperfections, well, everything else started to make sense... I don't need to put myself or anyone else on a pedestal. Being who we are is amazing enough.

But then I still had to work on letting stuff go, and that is hard. Letting go of all those untruths we have been taught or subconsciously acquired. All the suffering we have been given by all the people who are also hurting but who didn't know a better way to handle themselves. All that stuff about "I must be perfect", comparisons and self-doubt! It took time, as I was addicted to self-doubt and striving to be a perfectionist. But, slowly, changes occurred, and continue to occur. I decided to choose compassion over the stories in my head...

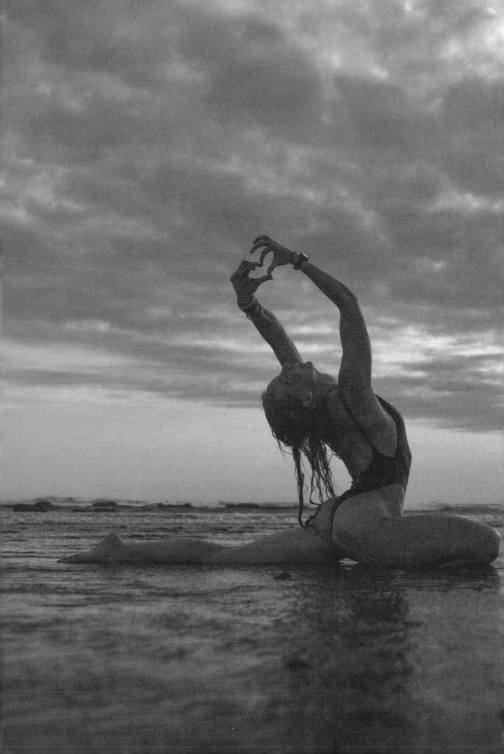

CHOOSING COMPASSION OVER STORIES IN OUR HEAD

CHAPTER 3:
CHOOSING COMPASSION OVER STORIES IN OUR HEAD

People often ask me how I keep fit. It's a great question, as many of us believe fitness means sticking to a rigid routine. To some extent, this is true, of course. Self-discipline is important. However, it's also important that this belief doesn't lead us to tell ourselves the false story that if we skip a day of training we will have somehow failed.

I have to miss many days for one reason or other. The key is that I just accept with compassion why I can't train on those days and show up the best I can, without worry, on all the other days. Otherwise, a sense of guilt or failure about just a few days might stop me showing up at all: an example of a story in my own head having the power to win over the truth and prevent me from achieving my goals.

Whether we know it or not, we tend to carry around untrue and unhelpful stories, and beliefs, in our heads about all sorts of things, including about ourselves. And, if we're not careful, these can hold us back in all sorts of ways. Yet it can be really hard to identify and unpick these stories. So how can we begin? In this chapter we'll explore a number of key concepts that I've found can help:

* **DETACHING FROM OUR EXPECTATIONS** – how liberating would it feel to simply embrace whatever emerged and enjoy each moment instead of being so caught up in "shoulds" and "shouldn'ts"?

* **QUIETENING OUR INNER CRITIC** – does a little nagging voice in your head tell you you're not quite good enough? How amazing would it be if we could learn to be less affected by this voice?

* **LETTING GO OF JUDGEMENT** – wouldn't the world be a nicer place to live if we could learn to just be kind to both ourselves and others, rather than looking for faults and weaknesses?

Once we learn to gently let go of all the unhelpful stories that we've been carrying around in our heads as if they're truths, we can turn the page and move into a new, more compassionate chapter of our lives.

DETACHING FROM OUR EXPECTATIONS

While it's great to have goals and to strive towards them, the more attachment we have in our own heads to any particular anticipated outcomes, the less satisfied we can be in the here and now if we're not careful. As such, expectations – whether set by ourselves or others – can end up causing a huge amount of pain and unhappiness.

LETTING GO OF OUTCOMES

One of the many things I love about yoga is that it teaches us to observe not just our bodies but also our minds without judgement or expectation – by grounding ourselves in the moment via breath and movement. This is something that I've been working on for a while in terms of expectations both on and off the mat! And it has helped me to go from constantly comparing myself with others, and getting caught up in my own and society's expectations (whether about how my body looks, how flexible I am in my yoga practice or how I deal with online haters), to finding a place where I don't need anything else to change – I just need to accept things as they unfold and "be".

This means I'm not distracted by trying to meet unrealistic expectations or control elusive results either in my yoga poses or beyond. I am instead free to simply enjoy the present moment.

LOOSENING THE CHAINS OF EXPECTATION

When I first became a mother, I had lost an unborn child the year before. It was heartbreaking. As a result, I set myself crazy parenting expectations and tried so hard to be the "perfect" mum that it nearly broke me. In the end, I realized that I was going to offer my daughter much more happiness if I simply followed what felt right to me in the moment, rather than running myself into the ground trying to fulfil lots of inherited expectations that felt like they were holding me prisoner. We are all more brilliant than we will ever realize, so it's time to forget about all the lurking "musts" and "shoulds" and embody the only thing we can be: ourselves. It's time to trust and believe in ourselves.

TURNING THE GAZE INWARDS

Many of us have become a new style of hunter in the world – hunters of external validation. It's time for the hunt to begin again, but this time with the gaze turned inwards – to our own hearts and souls – so that we no longer look externally for validation of our self-worth.

THE GIFT OF GRATITUDE

A seemingly simple but amazing way of freeing ourselves from the many stories in our head, including expectations, and connecting to our deeper sense of self-worth is to direct our attention to what we already have in life, instead of focusing on what we lack or want.

Like anyone else's, my life is far from perfect, but the gift of gratitude makes it beautiful. So, please repeat after me: Thank you! Thank you! Thank you! Thank you for everything I have and everything I am. We live in a wonderful world, full of magic and beauty as well as challenges. Full of sunsets, rainbows and smiles to enjoy. Full of birds singing, children laughing and hearts beating for our souls to dance to... If we focus only on the far distance, we might miss what's right in front of us. So let's be present, recognize and drop unhelpful expectations, give thanks and enjoy whatever comes: it's beautiful and so are you!

And if you find that compliment hard to take in, let's next consider how we might be able to quieten the voice of our inner critic in order to tune more into the beautiful music of the Universe around us...

QUIETENING OUR INNER CRITIC

Our inner critic is that little voice in our heads that tells us that we're not good enough, that we'll never be good enough no matter what we do. A voice of doubt, shame and self-blame. If we listen to it, it will keep us from finding our true purpose in the world. But, as hard as it is, we each have the power to quieten this inner critic. I know, as I've done it for myself, and I can't tell you how much happier I feel as a result.

WATCHING OUR THOUGHTS BLOW WITH THE WIND

It's said that we have fifty to sixty thousand thoughts every day, and that the ones that stress us the most are the ones we keep paying attention to – the ones we can't let go of, which are, unfortunately, often negative. Thoughts such as "I'm so useless", "I'm such a failure", "Why did I do that?" or "It's no big deal" (about something great we've just achieved). Such thoughts arrive like loud winds rattling the windows of our whole being.

It often feels like we only have two options: either open the windows to stop the rattling and let them cause chaos, or resist them by boarding up all the windows and get annoyed as they rattle all the louder. But there's a third option that we often forget about, and that's to just accept that the winds are there, rattling the windows (as that's what they do), and let them simply be.

The same approach can be taken when it comes to the challenging thoughts with which our inner critic bombards us. Yoga teaches us to remember that we can simply choose to sit in the moment and observe these thoughts passing, in the same way as we can watch clouds move through the sky.

DON'T MIND THE MIND

The goal is not to *silence* our inner critic, but simply to acknowledge that it's there, recognize when it's speaking, and remember that we don't have to listen to it when it won't help us.

And what's interesting is that when we stop paying it so much attention, its voice will naturally begin to quieten, allowing us to see the true essence of ourselves again, beneath the clouds.

THE THINGS OUR INNER CRITIC DOESN'T TELL US

It can be difficult to see the qualities in ourselves that other people like, admire and love; we're so often our own harshest critic. So let me remind you of some truths:

* *You are not a failure if you don't know the answer.*

* *You are not a failure if your body isn't model material.*

* *You are not a failure if your house is a bombsite.*

* *You are not a failure if you are divorced or not happily married.*

* *You are not a failure if you are a single mum or dad.*

* *You are not a failure if you eat fast food.*

* *You are not a failure if you're tired or forgetful.*

* *You are not a failure if you doubt yourself.*

* *You are not a failure if you have a bad day.*

* *You are not a failure.*

I want you to hear and really take in these truths, and the many more that follow from them. Please remember them the next time your inner critic's voice is getting louder and more persistent.

"DON'T MIND THE MIND — YOU ARE NOT YOUR THOUGHTS"

WE ARE ALL FRAGILE AND BEAUTIFUL INSIDE

It's easy to think at times that other people – whether the "popular girl" at school, that super-smart colleague, the flexible girl who does yoga online, or celebrities – don't experience the same kind of self-doubt (and, at times, maybe even self-loathing) as us. But everyone has an inner critic, no matter how popular, attractive, clever, rich, famous or whatever else. So it's just a matter of how much we each choose to listen to it and let it rule us, or not.

LIVING WITH UNCERTAINTY

Despite being aware of my inner critic and having worked hard at quietening it, I certainly don't yet have all the answers – I'm just a student of life, forever learning, trying, hoping, falling down and getting up again. Like everyone else, I'm learning to live with the many uncertainties, ups and downs of life.

Sometimes I feel like I'm a failure, and sometimes I know I can conquer the highest mountain. Sometimes I'm a mess inside even though I look like I've got it all together on the outside. Sometimes the critics cripple me, and sometimes their words hardly touch the sides. Sometimes I can live life with fierceness, and sometimes I don't want to get out of bed. But, through it all, I work on quietening the voice of my inner critic when I feel it trying to control me and keep me down with its negative commentary.

It is all a work in progress, but, on the whole, I try to let go of my judgements, be kind to myself and choose me over my negative thoughts. One method that I have found to help with this is to befriend my inner critic when its voice starts to dominate, so if you like this idea, please feel free to try the exercise overleaf.

BEFRIENDING YOUR INNER CRITIC

It might at first seem counterintuitive to befriend our inner critic when it's generally not something that we want to play a big role in our lives, but, ironically, in my experience, if we can learn to acknowledge it, without acting on it, the voice will start to lose its power.

1. Choose a time when you won't be distracted for a few moments. Let your thoughts rise like bubbles, floating to the surface of your mind without judgement.

2. If you hear the negative voice of your inner critic starting up, respond to it as you would a visitor, from a detached and neutral perspective. For example: "Here's my inner critic again. Hi there."

3. As negative thoughts arise, ask yourself whether you would allow anyone to speak to your five-year-old self in this way. If you wouldn't let your younger self go through this, then why let your inner critic get away with talking to your *current* self in this way?

4. Thank your inner critic for trying its best to look out for you and keep you safe, and reassure it that you're okay.

5. If the pronoun "I" appears in any of its fault-finding thoughts (such as "I don't know why I bother training at all as I so often don't make it onto my yoga mat"), try turning it around by replacing the "I" with "you" and saying something positive, such as: "The fact that you didn't get on your yoga mat today doesn't mean you're a failure." (This is a research-tested technique called "self-distancing".)

6. Spend a few moments thinking about how you could reframe your inner critic's commentary to make it into an opportunity for you. For example, you might decide that the next time you're tempted to miss a yoga session, you'll check in with yourself to see if it's *definitely* not possible to make it onto the mat, with a little extra effort.

7. Finally, try replying to your inner critic's hurtful comments with a positive affirmation. As you breathe deeply, repeat to yourself: "I am enough just as I am."

While you're unlikely ever to become best friends with your inner critic, with a little practice, you might just make its voice a little quieter and a little less toxic.

LETTING GO OF JUDGEMENT

We live in a world where we constantly feel judged in all sorts of ways, whether for our school grades, our performance at work, our social interactions, our appearance, our fitness levels and all else. But what does all this judgement serve other than ultimately making some people feel temporarily good about themselves and a lot of other people feel bad or "not enough"?

JUDGEMENT DRAINS OUR ENERGY

Do we really want to spend our one precious life judging, criticizing and shaming ourselves and others? The answer for me is no. If I only have this one life, why would I waste energy on a mindset that puts people in boxes, hurts people, and destroys opportunities and possibilities?

Yoga teaches us that judgement – both of ourselves and others – is one of the primary signs of an anxious ego. By consciously bringing our awareness to judgement, we can begin to expose the unconscious negative patterns that lie at the root of it – our innermost worries and insecurities – and hopefully change them. Feelings of insecurity and unworthiness tend to create the biggest bullies and the saddest souls.

CAN WE UNLEARN JUDGEMENT?

At some point I learned to judge and criticize. For example, at some point I learned that cellulite should be hidden, that wrinkles aren't something to be proud of and that stretch marks made me less beautiful. At some point we all learned this kind of rubbish about how we, and others, are not enough. But the good news is that this means we can also *unlearn* it if we are willing to make the effort to do so.

TAKING RESPONSIBILITY

It can be easy to sit here blaming the world around us for having planted false beliefs and judgements in our heads, but at some point we have to say, "Hang on a minute, I decided to believe in all this too." Once we take responsibility in this way for the role that we ourselves have played in the decision to make judgement after judgement as we move through our days, and once we decide to make a change, we make the call to lead a life of love and compassion over fear and judgement. It's a big call, but a call that will change your life.

THE JUDGEMENT CYCLE

I grew up watching people trying so hard to fit in that they were willing to hide their true selves, yet they were judged anyway. So I decided to try to break the judgement cycle that I was stuck in by marching to the beat of my own drum after my suicide attempt. Today, I am so tired of judgement and shaming – both through my own experiences of it and seeing so many loved ones going through similar things.

It's fascinating to me that even in the world of yoga, where people so openly talk about the need for love, compassion, authenticity and healing, people are often stuck in their own heads, continuing to criticize and shame one another based on outdated beliefs and misplaced judgements – in my case mainly for what I wear, or don't wear, and how I choose to express myself through my body.

We all have a body, of course, but apparently it is only acceptable to some people if we dress and present it in a certain way that pleases them. To me, this approach is not true yoga, as it does not embrace acceptance and non-judgement. And, for my daughter's sake, for my sake, for all our sakes, I no longer want to be a part of this toxic cycle of judging and being judged.

"CHOOSE LOVE, NOT JUDGE- MENT"

WAKING UP TO THE WAYS WE JUDGE

It can feel hard to acknowledge just how much judgement we cast in our lives – both on ourselves and others. And it can feel really tough at times to break this cycle of judgement that we've fallen into. But it's an essential step to living braver, more beautiful lives.

If we can start listening to the love, kindness and compassion in our hearts rather than the false stories and fears in our heads, everything will become clear. There is no need to exhaust ourselves with expectations. And there is no need to hurt ourselves through incessant judgement. We have this one life, blessed souls, so please let's use it wisely!

Once we're able to let go of judgements and simply notice and enjoy things without expectation, we'll be free again to see things in the same way as young children do – with a renewed sense of innocence, curiosity and pure joy.

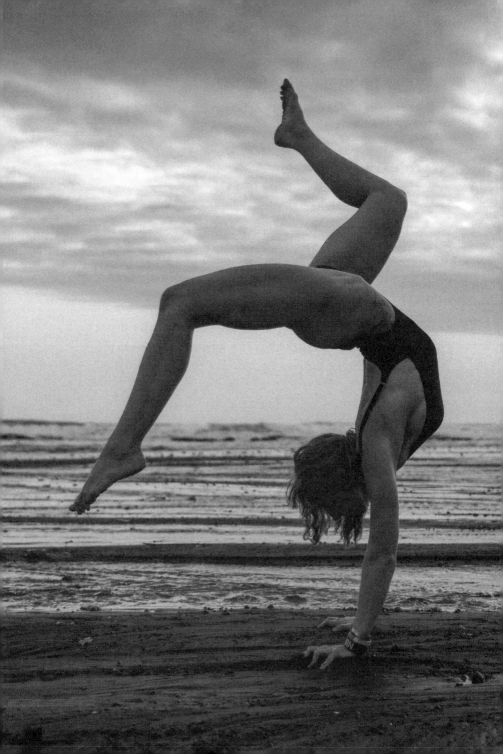

FREEING OUR INNER CHILD

CHAPTER 4:
FREEING OUR
INNER CHILD

Inside each of us is an inner child – a part of our innermost authentic self that got hidden at some point on the journey towards adulthood. This is the self that has the capacity to react to the world with a young child's spontaneity, openness, energy, candidness, courage, passion, joy, vulnerability and so much more. It is also the part of ourself that often carries any childhood hurt we experienced and that is the keeper of all the early lessons we learned about life.

At some point in our development, we unconsciously learned fear and anxiety, and started questioning our own perceptions. We therefore also started checking, and limiting, our choices and behaviours in line with this. Maybe it seemed, for example, that we had to be a certain way to be loved – whether clever, sporty, funny, "nice", a people-pleaser, or whatever else. Maybe we "learned", therefore, that a life of true love was an impossible fairytale.

But the good news is that our untarnished inner child is not lost; it is merely hidden beneath all this conditioning. So all we have to do to rediscover its magic, beauty and innocence is keep stripping away at the layers of negativity to "bare it all". In this chapter, we'll explore some of the key stages in this process of freeing our inner child:

✶ LEANING INTO NOT KNOWING – how liberating would it feel to return to a state of openness and curiosity, where we can flow with the changes rather than always feeling a need to be right?

✶ LETTING THE JOY BACK IN – wouldn't it be wonderful to have more fun and feel lighter in life, enjoying the unfiltered joy and wonder that we so often see in children?

✶ ALLOWING OURSELVES TO BE VULNERABLE – how much more authentic and free would we feel if we didn't think we had to hide our vulnerabilities as weaknesses? What if we could instead trust people to view them, and treat us, with pure love and compassion?

Our inner child reminds us that it's okay to be uncertain, to be silly, to play, to explore, to question, to make mistakes, to dance like no one's watching, to fall down, to get back up again and to adventure.

When we free our inner child, we also empower ourselves to heal emotional wounds from the past. And by doing this, we will end up bringing more love, light, beauty and courage not only into our own lives but also to those around us and the wider world.

LEANING INTO NOT KNOWING –
IT LETS US FIND OUT!

The unconscious conditioning that we undergo as we move through life means that, on the whole, we're programmed to look for certainties. We try to create order out of chaos in order to feel safe and on solid ground. Yet learning to be more accepting of when we don't know the answers to everything, as was the case when we were blank slates as children, can offer amazing opportunities for creativity and growth.

LOOSENING OUR GRIP ON THINGS

Many of us spend our days trying to do a million things at once: planning, worrying, procrastinating, expecting, predicting – the list goes on. But if we could just lift the pressure from ourselves and take things more as they come, without feeling a need to control every aspect, we could experience a whole lot more space and lightness.

TAKING LIFE ONE STEP AT A TIME

My main goal as a mum these days is simply to help my daughter, Laine, live her best life each day. That could mean Minnie Mouse before breakfast and who knows what after kindergarten. This means being open to taking the day one step at a time, not knowing quite what's going to come next and simply going with the flow.

In all these small daily moments, my heart realizes that I have everything I need and I am enough as I am, without knowing more, without planning more, without doing more – as when I look into my daughter's eyes, I find the purest love on earth.

THE COURAGE OF NOT KNOWING

This precious time with my daughter is a great reminder that bravery and beauty are not found in certainties and absolutes. They are found in the moments of openness and possibility, when we get a chance to use our creativity, our playfulness, our compassion, our patience, our tenacity, our strength of character, and just go for it!

And this applies to all situations, whether we are faced with a particularly tough task at work, dealing with the loss of a loved one, or in the midst of an existential crisis of some sort.

We can never know for sure what the future holds in any aspect of our lives, but it will come to meet us anyway. And I've learned that the key to not becoming completely lost and overwhelmed is to lean into all the uncertainty with love instead of fear.

CHOOSING LOVE OVER FEAR

It seems to me that love and fear are the key emotions that hold the power to allow our souls either to soar or to nose-dive. Fear wraps our bodies in chains and restricts us to a life of limiting beliefs. While love allows us to stand naked in our truth, giving us a chance to pass through pain to our greatest purpose. Fear attacks; love heals. Fear is about a threat that has not yet come to pass; love is the magical potential of each moment. Fear is division and separation; love is connection and unity.

THE ONLY CONSTANT IS CHANGE

It's amazing to think that our world can be changed by what we do in each and every moment. We can make a difference to the course of our day, our week, our year or maybe even our whole life in just a matter of seconds through our choices and actions. While it's

"STEP THROUGH FEAR INTO [FREEDOM]"

tempting to play it safe and stick to what we know, old hurts and fears will never be healed, and we will never really grow and flourish, if we continue to live in the shadow of the past.

When I take my fitness photos, I use a 10-second timer. It has taught me something very valuable. In those 10 seconds, everything can change. In 10 seconds, I can go from having the worst day to the best day, or vice versa. In 10 seconds, 42 babies are born in the world, and about 36 people die. So while a matter of seconds might not seem like a lot, they can be life-altering if we welcome them and the potential transformation they bring with a childlike openness and love. You don't need to go looking for miracles; you yourself are the miracle.

FiNDiNG FREEDOM

If we can manage to become aware of and put a stop to our fixed views of what we *think* we know about ourselves, and the world around us, we will realize that we're never as stuck in life as we might think we are. As even if we can't change our external circumstances, we can always change our internal perspectives. And if we can change this, we can change everything.

So let's reconnect with our inner child, lean into not knowing and create space to explore and play more. The exercise overleaf encourages you to do exactly this, so please feel free to try it any time you could do with a little light relief in life.

IT'S TIME TO PLAY AGAIN

As we move from childhood to adulthood, we can forget the joy that lies in the simple art of playing, when the focus is on just enjoying an experience rather than getting caught up in results. Maybe it's time to give ourselves permission to play again? If you like this idea, try the steps below.

1. Take a pen and some paper or a notebook to a quiet space where you will not be disturbed for a few minutes.

2. Enjoy a few, long, relaxed breaths as you check in with yourself.

3. When you are ready, think back to a time in your childhood when you felt really happy. What were you doing? And who were you with?

4. Write down all the details that you can remember about this time: the setting, people, activities, smells, colours, feelings...

5. Now let your memory wander back to other childhood memories that made your heart come alive and jot down those experiences too.

6. There's no limit to the amount you can write, so just continue until you feel like stopping. Then take a moment to read through your list.

7. How do you feel reading what you have written?

8. As you consider them all, are there any common features that connect the experiences? Certain people, places, activities or anything else?

9. If so, might there be ways that you could bring those aspects back into your life today? Maybe by finding out about evening art or dance classes? Taking singing lessons? Joining a local team?

10. Be sure to investigate all the possibilities in order to set your inner child free again.

Letting your inner child guide you in this way will lead you to the place where your happiness lies and where you will experience pure joy again.

LETTING THE JOY BACK IN

We were all born to play and explore, to dance to the beat of our heart, to roam free with the innocence of a child and the spirit of untamed horses. So I wish you a million ways of letting this kind of joy back into your life, so that you can once again experience the feeling of laughing without hesitation, living without limits and loving like it's all there is.

EXPLORING WHAT LIGHTS US UP

When I hit my lowest point after my suicide attempt, I was lucky enough to reconnect with my inner child when I started exploring the art of yoga handstands. Who could have ever have predicted that it would be this random activity that would end up being such a turning point in my life? I guess because I was upside down a lot of the time, my frown slowly turned into a natural smile!

But, as well as learning how to do handstands, I read books that touched my heart, soul and mind; I gave myself permission to dress up nicely and take myself out somewhere special – just because. And I danced in my living room to music that I loved any chance I got. The combination of doing all these things that I *used* to love before life got so tough and I had fallen into depression slowly started letting me see some chinks of light in the darkness.

BUILDING A RECONNECTION TOOLKIT

Some days I still feel sad, lonely or lost, but I now know that the seemingly simple acts of connecting with my breath and body, getting upside down, goofy dancing and even dressing up and treating myself to something nice can help me at least a little! It's my wish for you that you can get to know what your equivalent reconnection tools are in life so that there are at least some small things you can do to tap into your contented, naked core when dark days come along.

FINDING OUR OWN PATH THROUGH

It might be certain colours that help you feel calm or certain scents that uplift you. It might be watching a feel-good movie or singing at the top of your lungs to a song you first learned as a teenager. It might be having a bath and listening to classical music. It might be calling a friend or it might be going out for a walk in beautiful nature. It doesn't matter what it is, as long as it's something positive that could help you.

At times, of course, even activities that we know can make our heart soar may not help lift us out of a slump if we're feeling too numb or sad to feel into them and really enjoy them. But this doesn't mean there's no point in doing them. It just means we may need to keep repeatedly doing them, with a sense of trust that our joy and spark will return in the end. I'm still learning to make things awesome for myself. I now accept that it's a life-long work in progress for us all.

MOVING OUR BODIES

For me, movement is freedom: the more I move, the freer I feel both internally and externally. It's as though I come home to myself and my body, and move away from all the unhelpful stories and attachments that no longer serve me. Like anyone else, I get affected by the labels, judgements and expectations that land at my door. However, movement allows me to transition through it to a place of heartfelt joy – where I remember that all we really need to be at peace is to be who we are right here and now, fully and without apology.

As a result, I now dance my way through each day not because of any music but because I have found the true beat of my own heart – and the rhythm of life within myself.

So why not explore the art of movement for yourself? You may not find a love for yoga, handstands, dancing and physical workouts as I have, but you may instead find a love for something completely different, whether walking, running, football, gymnastics, roller blading or any of the other myriad possibilities out there that allow us to connect with and truly appeciate our body and breath.

SIMPLIFYING THINGS

If time is in short supply to explore what activities bring you most joy, it can be useful to take stock of your priorities in life in order to simplify things to free up dedicated time for yourself.

Set aside 10–15 minutes when you'll be undisturbed and have a think about what the most important things to you are in life. Write these down, read them back to yourself and assess whether you are actually devoting time to these activities. For example, are you spending time with your friends and family? Are you spending time outside, soaking up the sun and dancing in the rain? Are you spending time learning new things or helping others? If so, great! But if not, then it's time to change things so that you are...

DON'T SWEAT THE SMALL STUFF

Once we know what's most important to us at the core, it will be easier to avoid worry and stress by letting less significant things slide.

I realized as I was writing this book that another useful way for me to think about this was in the form of what key snippets of life advice I would give my daughter when I feel she's old enough. So see the list opposite for my initial draft of this. No doubt I will fine-tune it as life unfolds around us, but for now it acts as a useful compass for me to open my heart to as much love and joy as I can in my life.

10 THINGS I WILL TELL MY DAUGHTER TO DECREASE HER STRESS AND ENHANCE HER JOY

1. You are not any one thing; you are a beautiful, multi-faceted human, full of all kinds of awesomeness.

2. If the world tries to put labels on you, know it's not about you; it's about the world. We are all perfect in our imperfection.

3. Love without reservation, and ask yourself: "Am I showing *myself* love too?"

4. When you get your heart broken – and it will happen, my love – remember that it will pass and the sun will soon come out again from behind the clouds.

5. If it's 3 a.m. and you still don't understand something, sleep it off.

6. When it rains, don't feel you have to wait for the storm to pass if you want to dance outside.

7. Never judge a book by its cover. The inside is what counts.

8. It is entirely acceptable to wear blue with green and pink with red. And to wear absolutely anything you want, in fact. Colour or cut your hair how you like. Wear bold makeup – or none at all. Anything goes. You are the master of your own destiny.

9. Life is short. Explore, play. Laugh, cry. Have seconds if you're hungry. And enjoy dessert – without guilt!

10. Always be authentic and truthful, open and gentle, accepting and compassionate. This will make you both beautiful and brave.

"LET YOUR VULNERA-BILITY UNLOCK YOUR POWER"

ALLOWING OURSELVES TO BE VULNERABLE

Professor Brené Brown talks of vulnerability as "the birthplace of love, belonging, joy, courage, empathy, and creativity". And I for one strongly identify with this: it's when I've been at my most vulnerable that I've had to dig deepest in order to find a way forward and grow.

BREAKING DOWN THE WALLS WE BUILD

Many of us build walls in our hearts and minds to protect ourselves from hurt, but if we're not careful these can become a self-imposed prison. As well as protecting us from potential harm, they can limit our space in which to blossom, so that we end up stuck and stagnating. Stepping out from these walls requires great courage as it means initially exposing ourselves to potential hurt and danger.

When I took the decision to start sharing so much of myself online, I was consciously stepping outside of my introvert comfort zone to make myself vulnerable, as, for me, vulnerability is an opportunity to connect with others, to learn and to grow. It is life at its most honest, when we own our truths, and it can be extremely healing to the world.

COMING HOME TO OURSELVES

Vulnerability can bring us to some challenging places. If you get lost on the path, let your inner child reach out its hand to guide you back home to yourself. The great Sufi poet Rumi reminds us: "Your task is not to seek love, but merely to seek and find all of the barriers within yourself that you have built against it." Love in the knowledge that love makes us vulnerable, and with vulnerability comes great authenticity, strength, power, bravery and beauty.

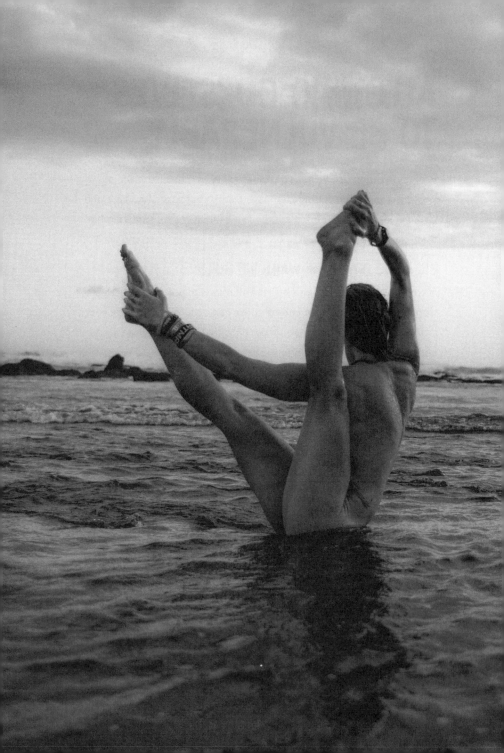

REALIZING DARKNESS ALLOWS OUR LIGHT TO SHINE

CHAPTER 5:

REALIZING DARKNESS ALLOWS OUR LIGHT TO SHINE

Just as there is both day and night, so we all naturally have a balance of both light and dark within us. When I made the attempt on my own life in 2014, the darkness had taken me over. I felt that nobody was there for me, including myself, and that it would make no difference if I was gone. But it was this state of utter darkness that ultimately set me on the path to living in my own light again.

I'm not suggesting that everyone has to hit rock bottom before they can rise, but it's important to recognize that darkness and light coexist, and that dark times therefore aren't in themselves always a bad thing. After all, it's hard to see the flame of a candle on a sunny day, isn't it? It's only the darkness that allows the light to shine.

When I tell people I tried to commit suicide, I often get blank stares, shocked expressions and comments such as "You're joking, right?" as people feel overwhelmed by the idea. But instead of overwhelming us, darkness can – if viewed in a certain way – spur us on, moving us away from the "shoulds" and "musts" – towards the path less followed, of our individual truth. In this chapter, we'll explore several main ways in which we can learn to better deal with darkness in our lives:

✳ **ACCEPTING BOTH THE DARK AND THE LIGHT**
– do we, in trying to avoid dark, difficult times in our lives,
end up inadvertently denying ourselves the experience of
the brightest possible times too?

✳ **SEEING THE STRENGTH IN SURRENDERING** – how
much less stressful and more serene might our lives feel if we
could learn to trust and accept more, and resist and battle less?

✳ **LEARNING FROM THE SACRED CLOWNS (THE
HATERS)** – what if, instead of letting the people who challenge
and attack us get us down, we decided that it was better for us to
forgive them and look for lessons in their less-than-kind behaviour?

While we all contain elements of both light and dark, what matters
is how we manage the balance between the two and how we choose
to act on this. The first step, however, is simply acknowledging that
light and dark really do co-exist inside us all and that this is okay.

ACCEPTING BOTH THE DARK AND THE LIGHT – DROPPING RESISTANCE

When we resist something, we expend a lot of energy trying to block it and stop it from happening. However, sometimes negative thoughts, worries and fears – whether we're conscious of them or not – can cause forms of resistance that also deny us all sorts of amazing opportunities that are out there, waiting for us.

SHINING A LIGHT ON RESISTANCE

Resistance lurks in the dark corners of our psyche. For example, resistance to any form of potential risk or failure is often the knee-jerk reaction that makes us retreat when we're about to leap forwards; that prompts us to say, "I can't", "I shouldn't" and "I won't"; and that leads us to make excuses for not following our dreams.

By becoming aware of our own patterns of resistance, we already start to lessen its potential hold on us. Our life, heart and mind are full of shadows and always will be. But those shadows cannot withstand the patience and perseverance of light. So when you next feel a sense of resistance rising up and keeping you in the darkness of your doubts, fears and other negative thoughts, make a decision to shine your light on these things holding you back.

Our inner light is fed by the strength that we have accrued from the adversity, limits and darkness that we have already overcome. It comes from knowing that you have fallen down many times, but you have always got up again and you are still standing.

FROM DARKNESS INTO LIGHT

By shining a light of awareness, acceptance and non-judgement on any darkness that we feel within, we can start to see our negative thoughts, doubts, worries, fears and so on more clearly – for what they are, rather than what we have presumed them to be. And once we can see things more clearly, we often no longer fear them in the same way, which allows us to drop our resistance to them and instead just be aware of them and get on with things anyway. By confronting our darkness, we therefore light our own path to freedom.

PLAYING IN THE DARK

A while ago, when my inner demons reared their ugly heads again, I decided to take up pole dancing – something I had always been intrigued by. By playing and practising on my pole, I put myself in a safe place where I could step into the darkness and gently explore what my demons had been feeding on. As I swung and hung and enjoyed the sense of being physically strong and alive, I confronted my demons, telling them that I love myself – that I'm enough. The thing about confronting chaos is that while it disturbs us, it also forces our hearts to roar in ways we secretly find magnificent and inspiring.

So facing the darkness in our lives doesn't always have to be an oh-so-serious business. We can each find our own unique, light-powered and joy-filled strategies for tackling resistance. So what activities might you be up for exploring, getting lost in and using as a springboard for exploring your darker side?

BECOME THE LIGHT THAT SPARKS THE FLAME

The world doesn't need more people talking about what they *hope* to do, or thinking about what they *should* be doing. The world needs more people coming alive. It needs us to overcome our resistance

"LET YOUR LIGHT SHINE LIKE A STAR"

and live the brave, beautiful, joyous and magical lives we were meant to lead. When we do this, our light will give other people permission and inspiration to shine, too. They'll see you and think, "Oh, maybe I can do that too!"

When this happens, we are triggering people to feel what they need to feel in order to grow out of their smallness, limiting beliefs, destructive behaviours and darkness – and into their own light! So own your awesomeness and your successes. Everyone benefits when you do. We are a collective and we have the power to lift each other up – and to shine like stars together.

SHARING OUR LIGHT

When I was at my lowest, the darkness called depression said to me: "You are broken from the inside." Troubling thoughts flooded my head the whole time and it was hard to know what was real and what wasn't. If left unchecked, this kind of darkness can devour us, as almost happened to me. As such, some people sadly never get the chance to shift their resistance into acceptance, their darkness into light, their pain into joy.

When we look up at the stars, we don't know which ones are still alive, their light just not yet having fully faded. We don't know which ones are already dead on the inside. People are like that as well. I was like that once too. So if you see someone struggling to show their own light, floundering in the darkness or resisting all that is good in life, please don't judge them or have the attitude of "Oh, he or she will be all right – it'll pass". Connect to those you love, call them, sit with them, allow space for them, accept them as they are, tell them you love them (darkness 'n' all), tell them again, and again – and shine your light on them. You could save a life.

SEEING THE STRENGTH IN SURRENDERING

The word "surrender" is often associated with weakness in the sense of giving up on something because we are losing. But surrender can also be a hugely empowering tool when we find ourselves in circumstances beyond our control – a gateway to trust, freedom and growth.

LETTING GO OF OUR NEED TO CONTROL

Sometimes, no matter what we do or how hard we try, things just don't work out the way we planned. Some days I kick ass, but, to be honest, most days life kicks *me* in the ass. Some days I stand up again, but many days I just have to sit for a while, wondering how on earth to get up. Life isn't easy, but I would not have it any other way, because it's teaching me to show up for myself and my daughter.

Watching her learn to walk, talk and all the rest has been reminding me that falling on our ass now and again is, of course, a natural part of growth – so while I'm down there I might as well accept it, surrender myself to it and enjoy sliding, spinning, smiling and laughing before I get back up and try again!

SURRENDERING TO THE FLOW

Life isn't made to fit into neat, labelled boxes. We humans are all beautiful, flawed, multi-faceted souls who are elemental, primal and fluid like water. So let's surrender to this and allow our lives to flow!

Let's not cage ourselves in by trying to control every little detail, and then call that living. When we stop trying to exert control, we surrender, adapt and grow – and that is how we uncover the hidden beauty of ourselves. So let's see the strength in this!

LETTING GO OF REGRETS

Please stop worrying about getting back to who you were before things "all went wrong". To heal and be the true definition of strength, bravery and beauty is to understand that the person you have become, and are becoming, is the soul who is most capable of doing whatever it is that you were put here on earth to do.

That you've changed isn't a critical statement – because change is as natural as the passing seasons. From the darkness of winter, the earth emerges blooming in spring. From the brightness of summer, the earth slips into the raging colours of autumn. From here, it cools into a quieter state of winter where everything seems still – but beneath the grey skies the earth is resting and rejuvenating, ready to bloom again. Surrender means trust. Trust in ourselves, trust in the Universe, trust that truth and love will slowly emerge.

SURRENDERING TO THE TRUTH OF OUR EMOTIONS

Try not to hate your tears of rebirth, your painful fractures of re-growth. These broken pieces form the fragments of a bright new mosaic, waiting to be pieced together into a thing of beauty.

You will be surprised by how amazing everything becomes as you embrace and merge with the new person you are becoming, instead of feeling overwhelmed by all that you have been through.

It is in digging through the chaos, dancing in the thunder, piecing ourselves together bit by bit in all our newfound glory, that we will find a whole new level of happiness, courage, strength, tenderness, fresh possibilities and love – and we can then surrender into that.

The Child's Pose exercise overleaf will offer you a *physical* experience of surrender in preparation for allowing more *emotional* surrender into your life.

GIVE YOURSELF TO CHILD'S POSE

In yoga, we often talk about letting go and surrendering ourselves to poses. Child's Pose (*Balasana* in Sanskrit) is a wonderful position to relax the body and quieten the mind, but really allowing yourself to surrender into it will bring all the more physical and mental release.

1. Kneel on an exercise mat or carpet, and focus on your breath. Allow your attention to turn inwards.

2. Enjoy a couple of deep, relaxing inhales and exhales, letting your breath lengthen.

3. Spread your knees apart while keeping your big toes touching. Rest your behind on your heels.

4. On an exhale, fold forward so that your chest rests between or (if your legs are together) on top of your thighs. Rest your forehead on the mat while you lay your arms alongside your body, palms up.

5. Close your eyes.

6. Feel how the tension in your back begins to drain away.

7. Sense the air entering and leaving your lungs, and let yourself relax more deeply into the pose with each exhale. Hold this position for a minute or two.

8. When you are ready, sit back upright on your heels before resuming your everyday activities.

Child's Pose can be a great way to start and end each day as it helps to create a feeling of calm and safety.

Caution: Please do not attempt Child's Pose if you have knee problems. And pregnant women should avoid resting their belly on their thighs.

LEARNING FROM THE SACRED CLOWNS (THE HATERS)

Sacred clowns are figures that have featured in ancient cultures around the world, challenging the normal order of things and creating chaos and anarchy. In my own life, as hard as it can be at times, I like to think of the online trolls and others who are quick to judge and criticize me as serving a similar purpose – challenging me to meet their words and actions with courage, compassion, love and respect.

MY EXPERIENCE OF SACRED CLOWNS

As I've mentioned already, when I share photos and videos of myself online, many people choose to cast less than favourable judgements on how I present myself. Some accuse me of creating yoga-inappropriate content, others sexually gratifying content. And some of my images have even been misappropriated and used by a number of people for their own sexualized purposes, which breaks my heart.

BEING BRAVE AND BARING IT ALL

I respect my body and the skin I am in – just as I respect everyone else's. Being an Aussie and a swimmer, I grew up in swimsuits. These days, I don't think twice about wearing a bikini, or possibly less. It's just who I am. I was taught I am only borrowing my body for my soul's home in this lifetime, and that my life experience is shaped by how I use my body, not by what it wears.

In Europe, I can go into a sauna naked with strangers, and we'll sit and have a conversation like people in any other normal situation.

Yet if I post a swimsuit or an underwear photo on social media, suddenly I'm labelled everything from a woman of little virtue and a porn star to an individual undeserving of respect and a bad mother.

In the same way, I can be on the beach in a bikini, yet if I wear a short skirt in the street, I might be questioned about whether I'm setting a good example for my daughter.

Less clothing doesn't make anyone a bad person or hurt anyone. Yet it hurts me deeply every time someone puts a label on me when they don't even know me and what I stand for.

WHY THE SHAMING?

How is it that humans can judge and hate so much? In my opinion, the answer is actually pretty simple: it's because, on the whole, most people are, sadly, living from a place of fear, separation and ultimately darkness – rather than from a place of acceptance, love and light! As such, many of us live in fear of what's different or unfamiliar.

But why is there so much shame – and shaming! – around the incredible human body in particular? And why is it that when someone reveals their body in all its beautiful glory, so many people see it in a sexual way, are threatened or offended by it, get defensive and feel the need to judge, make assumptions and criticize?

I believe the answer to these questions is that, deep down, these things resonate with an issue that people have about *themselves* and their own bodies – based on their own limiting learned beliefs and perceptions. As I see it, nothing external could have the ability to challenge people this much unless they feel unstable about the topic within themselves – which is where the chance to learn emerges.

So maybe it's time to stop asking what's wrong with *other* people, their choices and behaviours, and instead start asking ourselves what we need to change in society so that innocent things like nudity and choice of clothing no longer carry the stigma and power to make people act from a place of shame and fear – and instead give cause for joy and celebration.

Maybe it's time to question how it could have got to the point that women's bodies have been so overtly objectified and sexualized over the years that women are now hating on other women for how they choose to present themselves – rather than supporting and applauding them for reclaiming their own bodies, baring their authentic selves and celebrating the human body in all its glory, whether clothed or naked?

OWNING OUR CHOICES

Clothing does not define us or determine our value. Neither does age, body shape, skin colour, physical ability, mental ability, line of work, gender, sexual preference, family background, relationship status, number of followers on social media, bank balance or any other number of things. Only we, ourselves, get to choose who we are.

Clothing or the lack thereof is a form of self-expression. We are all responsible for our own comfort and individuality. So please feel free to wear what makes you happy, and I'll wear what makes me happy.

NO MORE PEOPLE-PLEASING, PLEASE!

The mean comments I receive on social media often challenge me to feel bad about myself. Even though I usually get at least five positive comments for every negative – and I am sooooo very appreciative of all the amazing positive interactions – the negative ones often tend to hit home the most strongly.

I've thought about this a lot, trying to figure out why it's the case, and I've come to the realization that it's because I've learned, without knowing it, throughout my life to be what is often known as a "people pleaser". When we people-please, we go out of our way to make *others* happy. We avoid confrontation and find it hard to say no, as we hate even the *idea* of others being critical of us or feeling unhappy. Yet the truth is that people-pleasing robs us of a little of ourselves each time we do it, as it's not coming from the core of our true, authentic self; it's all about masks and show.

All the "sacred clowns" in my life have therefore helped me develop the courage to accept that it's okay to be misunderstood, disliked or excluded. And this very acceptance – and the forgiveness of the haters that comes with it – has the power to set me free and save me from my own darkness.

Even though it might feel at times as if we're alone in the dark, when we are honest and true to ourselves, we become the light that guides the way.

FOCUSING ON THE LOVERS, NOT THE HATERS

Remember: as many haters as there are in the world – operating from a place of fear and judgement – there are just as many, if not more, who will see our magic right away. And these are the people to focus on and spend our time with.

These people will make us feel like we can be even *more* ourselves, not less. They will hold space for us and want to know how our hearts are. They will treat us with love, compassion and respect – and they will help us shine our light even brighter and live the life of incredible love that both we and they deserve.

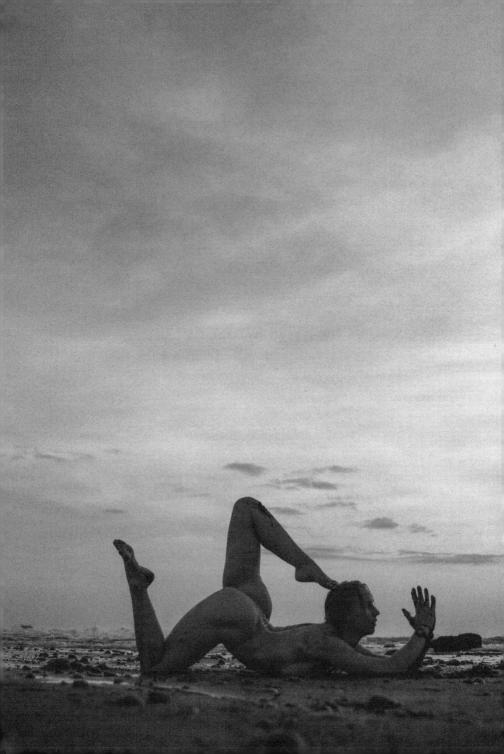

EMBRAC-ING OUR INNATE SENSUAL-ITY

CHAPTER 6:
EMBRACING OUR INNATE SENSUALITY

I've always been taught that our bodies are simply the vehicles that we have been gifted for our souls to interact with the physical world in all its wonder. As such, in and of itself, the human body is a neutral space. Any labels assigned to it – whether "beautiful", "sexy", "sensual" or whatever else – come from the society in which we live.

Having said that, as a vehicle for our physical experiences, there's no denying that our bodies have an innate – and what some might call divine or God-given – sensuality, by which I mean a natural ability to fully experience, express and enjoy our physical senses – seeing, hearing, smelling, tasting, touching and feeling – for optimal physical pleasure, as well as for optimal everyday functioning. Anyone fully in touch and at ease with the wide spectrum of their sensuality therefore has the capacity to live a life that feels both supremely fulfilling and supremely free.

Unfortunately, there is often a lot of confusion between the notion of sensuality and sexuality, which has led to us being encouraged to temper our "sensuality" for fear of coming across as too "bold", "brazen", "inappropriate"... (the list goes on). There is, however, immense value in understanding and connecting with our divine sensuality, so in this chapter we will explore several aspects of this:

✳ THE RELATIONSHIP BETWEEN SENSUALITY AND SEXUALITY – both sensuality and sexuality are part of the rich fabric of life, so how liberating would it feel to become more familiar with these aspects of ourselves without fear of judgement or shaming?

✳ RECLAIMING OUR OWN BODIES AND BEAUTY – isn't it time that we defined for *ourselves* what makes us feel sensual, brave and beautiful in this world, rather than being restricted by the limited or outdated opinions of others?

✳ VALUING BOTH FEMININE AND MASCULINE ENERGY – instead of expecting ourselves to be just one thing or another, how amazing might it feel to celebrate the immense value of both our soft yin side *and* our more intense yang side?

Embracing our divine and innate sensuality means being entirely comfortable with *all* aspects of our own bodies and beings – radiating confidence without needing other people's approval. What could be more brave and beautiful than that?

THE RELATIONSHIP BETWEEN SENSUALITY AND SEXUALITY

As explored on the previous page, sensuality – the experience, expression and enjoyment of physical pleasures – lies at the root of who we are as human beings. As spiritual souls living in physical bodies, sensuality comes into existence the moment our hearts begin beating and our breath starts its rhythmic course, inviting us to join the dance of life. Equally, sexuality – the combination of our sexual feelings, thoughts, attractions and behaviours – is a fundamental part of who we are based on the fact that the very act of sexual intercourse is what brings us all into this amazing world in the first place.

DIFFERENTIATING BETWEEN THE TWO

There's no doubt, of course, that our sensuality and sexuality are linked: when we are fully awakened to our senses and sensuality – which can manifest in all sorts of ways in each of our lives – it can contribute greatly to our sense of sexual connection and sexuality.

It's important, however, to recognize that sensuality and sexuality are not one and the same. For example, sexuality can exist without sensuality when it's based purely on the more animalistic responses of the human body, as is often prevalent in the porn industry – and sometimes also in more mainstream media. And if this is all that some of us are presented with as a notion of "sensuality", then it's no wonder that we can end up feeling uncomfortable about, or even ashamed of, our own, and others', sensual instincts, desires and needs.

RECONNECTING TO THE SELF

For me, sensuality is a way of being. After I experienced the traumas of sexual abuse and sexual assault in my early twenties, I went through a period where, sadly, I felt completely numb, joyless and disconnected from my body, as if I had been robbed of my senses.

As I worked to rediscover myself and start feeling something again, I found that – as well as feeding my soul by spending time in beautiful nature, surrounding myself with kind people and reading nourishing books – one of the best ways to re-establish a sense of meaningful connection with myself and my senses was physical movement, in my case mainly through yoga and pole dancing.

FINDING INNER FREEDOM

Something about the level of body awareness required to practise the postures and sequences, coupled with the amount of both self-expression and freedom of movement that the physical activities gave me, allowed me to get out of my head and back into a more sensual experience of life. For the first time in years, I felt truly liberated and alive again. Like a goddess in my own skin – able to recognize and undo all the conditioning and unhelpful labelling that had threatened to box me in – and the paralyzing fear that this had instilled in me. Little by little, I started to find the authentic core of who I was again – through the vehicle of my own body and breath.

REDEFINING PLEASURE

The more time I carved out to spend on these physical activities that I loved, the more pleasure I experienced in even the most mundane of activities and interactions. The greatest "pleasure" in life therefore no longer necessarily had to be sexual, as often implied, but instead could lie in the passion and sensuality that can be found in *any* activity.

"STAND TALL AND BLOSSOM LiKE A LOTUS"

OUR RELATiONSHiP WiTH NUDiTY

Choosing to view sensuality simply as a practice that can amplify the magic all around us that we so often feel disconnected from – rather than as something implicitly sexual – means that seeing images of people in the nude, such as a lot of my own online material, would in no way need to seem sexually "inappropriate", "provocative", "dirty", "offensive" or any of the other labels that are often aimed at me.

As it is, however, the human body has become sexualized to a confusing extent. Why, for example, are nipples, vaginas and some child-birth related images censored in many places? These things create and sustain life, yet society has twisted the truth so beautifully that we think we may somehow damage lives by showing them!?

Our conditioning within this context means it can be really difficult to feel comfortable enough to "bare it all". Yet, a naked body is the most natural thing that there is; we were all born this way, after all. So wouldn't it be amazing to just relax, honour and embrace this?

SENSUALiTY AS A FORM OF VULNERABiLiTY

It's important to be aware that, while connecting with our own sensuality is one of the most beautiful feelings in the world, choosing to lay this bare for others, whatever that might mean to each of us, brings with it a certain vulnerability – as other people may or may not view our form of sensual self-expression as "appropriate" within their own spheres of thinking.

But, just like a lotus flower, which rises and blossoms from darkness and mud, so too will we only truly blossom into the fully sensual beings we were born to be if we are able to accept and move through this sense of vulnerability. Only through knowing the pain that this can bring will we learn to be more understanding, compassionate, brave and beautiful within ourselves.

RECLAIMING OUR OWN BODIES AND BEAUTY

As already touched on, it's never the human body that is in itself ugly, offensive, flawed, "too this", "not enough that". It's only ever our own conditioned thoughts and opinions – and those of others – that create the stigmas. So isn't it time we reclaimed our bodies for ourselves by stopping these unhelpful thoughts from ruling the roost?

RECLAIMING OUR THOUGHTS

Change our thoughts and we can watch our life change before our eyes; change our thoughts and we can watch our body change, too, if we want. We can make a heaven out of hell, or a hell out of heaven, all by the way we think. If we want to feel more loved, let's change our thoughts. Want to feel more beautiful? Let's change our thoughts.

So let's stop hiding, berating and shaming ourselves. Instead, let's love and celebrate our bodies for all their glorious gifts. And let's spend our precious years on this planet thinking about something more worthwhile than our size, shape, weight and imaginary flaws!

THINK OUR BODIES BEAUTIFUL

Before I became pregnant, someone told me, "Don't have babies. Babies will ruin your body." And after I first gave birth and fell into post-natal depression, I thought that it had! But with the wisdom of hindsight I can now see, of course, that nothing but my own perspective has the power to ruin my body! And my perspective is now that my body is full of life. My body is fit and strong and powerful. My body gave me the chance to be a mother. If anything, I was ruined by the world before I knew my little girl, and she made me whole again.

AMAZING JUST AS WE ARE

I have one of the most sensitive skins. It took me a long time to get over this, as I was teased badly at school for being red-faced. It's not something that beauty magazines usually encourage us to aspire to! But red skin, acne, cellulite – whatever it is that you've got going on that you don't like about yourself – none of it need stop you from loving yourself and feeling proud to be you. It isn't a flaw. It's just you – being human.

So, please, let's stop our physical features from holding us back as a result of what society deems to be "beautiful", "sensual" or "sexy", and instead reclaim every aspect of our bodies for what they are: good enough and perfect as they are, as they're what we've got and we're lucky to have them.

I can't tell you the amount of times I'm reminded of my redness each day, but ultimately, it's just part of life. I can still be a mum, do a handstand and laugh, so really it means nothing. Similarly, you can have cellulite, excess fat, scars or whatever else, and still be a strong, healthy, kind, generous and generally wonderful human!

The likelihood is that if you saw a photo of yourself now in ten years' time, you'd be amazed at how gorgeous you were. So let's reclaim our own awesomeness and be amazed *now*! Let's celebrate ourselves and each other – whether red-faced or not, belly folds or not, cellulite or not. And let's not judge. But instead recognize "baring it all" in this way as the brave and beautiful act that it is.

LOVING OURSELVES AS WE LOVE OTHERS

We don't fall in love with someone just because they have a beautiful physical body. We might lust after them for this reason, but if they're not beautiful inside, it's unlikely to turn into lasting love. We fall in love with people's minds, souls, hearts, and the way they make us feel.

"THE WORLD NEEDS YOUR BEAUTY"

We find them beautiful because of how their body expresses these incredible inner qualities as part of their external being. So why treat ourselves any differently?

OWNiNG OUR OWN BEAUTY

In the past, I've taken photos of a zillion different poses to find a shot that makes me feel beautiful, but often nothing ever really succeeded. To be honest, I have never been considered conventionally beautiful. I have been called "cute", "goofy", "crazy", "blonde", "strong", "athletic", "flexible", "striking" and a million things in between. But "beautiful"? Not much...

However, I now realize, of course, that it isn't any pose or other external factor that will make me feel beautiful; it's the way I love myself, and the confidence that I have to be and "own" my authentic self – vulnerable but real.

THE BODY AS A WORK OF ART

We can admire physical perfection in the same way as we might admire a painting. However, like any art, the human body only becomes truly great when it makes us really *feel* something. So let's reclaim our bodies and all the sensuality that comes with that – and experience ourselves as the masterpieces that we were born to be!

If you'd like a little help with this, the exercise overleaf will show you how to work with your body's subtle energy system to feel more deeply connected and in flow.

UNBLOCKING YOUR SENSUAL ENERGY

It is believed in the yogic tradition that there are seven subtle energy centres in the body known as chakras. These begin at the base of the spine and ascend to the crown of the head, each one being linked with a different type of energy in the body. The second chakra up, known as the sacral chakra or *Svadhishthana*, is the one linked with creativity, flow, pleasure, sensuality, relationships and sexuality. If this chakra is underactive or blocked, you might find it difficult to get in touch with your sensuality, let go, express yourself and go with the flow in life. To help with this:

1. Sit quietly somewhere that you won't be disturbed for a few moments and take some deep, grounding breaths.

2. Place your hands on your lap, resting them on top of each other, with the palms facing up and thumbs touching.

3. Focus on the area of your spine at the height of your lower abdomen, which is where your sacral chakra is believed to be located.

4. Imagine this energy centre as the bud of a beautiful orange flower (orange is the colour traditionally associated with this chakra).

5. Think about the qualities linked with this chakra: creativity, flow, pleasure, sensuality, relationships and sexuality. Consider what they mean to you. As you do so, imagine the orange bud spiralling open, one petal at a time.

6. Silently and repeatedly chant the sound "Vam". (The vibrations of this sound traditionally linked to the sacral chakra are believed to cleanse and release any blockages.)

7. Continue to tune into the sacral chakra and observe any sensations that emerge, whether physical or emotional, until you feel ready to complete the meditation.

8. To finish, imagine the energy centre as a flower in full flourish and watch its petals gently close one by one.

9. When you are ready, gently return to your daily life.

Taking regular time out to connect with the energy of your sacral chakra in this way will help you to become more comfortable with, accepting of and willing to explore and express both your innate creativity and sensuality.

VALUING BOTH FEMININE AND MASCULINE ENERGY: YIN AND YANG

According to the ancient Chinese philosophy of Taoism, yin and yang are universal energies associated with feminine and masculine qualities (dark and light) that co-exist in everything and everyone. One cannot exist without the other, and each flows into the other in a constant state of flow. As such, each one of us, whatever our gender, is a beautiful, fluctuating balance of feminine and masculine energy.

EMBRACING HARMONY AND FLOW

The Taoist idea is that if we live in harmony with the principles of yin and yang, we start to go with the natural flow of the Universe, and our lives become much less of a struggle. And, while I'm by no means a practising Taoist, this fundamental principle makes complete sense to me as, if we were all able to accept both the feminine and masculine energies within ourselves, we'd see our inherent wholeness, just as we are, rather than falsely thinking that we're "not enough" and trying to force ourselves to be more this, more that, less this, less that...

THE YIN-YANG SYMBOL EXPLAINED

The visual symbol for yin and yang energy is a well-known one: a circle made of two interconnected swirls. The yin is the dark swirl, representing femininity, and the yang is the white one, representing masculinity. However, each also contains the seed of the other in the form of a small dot in the opposite colour – a visual clue as to just how interconnected they are believed to be. For instance, the trough of a wave is yin, whereas its crest is yang. Neither is better than the other; they are both simply aspects of the same wholeness.

BALANCiNG OUR ENERGiES

For many years, I wasted a lot of time and energy worrying about how "unfeminine" I felt. I always had a naturally slim body but it wasn't a particularly curvy one. And the more I got into my fitness, the leaner and more athletic I became – and the more "masculine" I felt. Add to this the sense of focus and intensity with which I tended to approach life, and rarely would I feel as if I was beautiful or womanly enough.

I now like to joke that as I'm "female", I'm the following combination: Fe = Iron; Male = Man. Therefore I'm an iron man! But the truth, if I take on the Taoist approach, is that I, like everyone else, contain an ever-changing balance of both feminine *and* masculine energies – neither right nor wrong in anyone of any gender; simply what it is and therefore worthy of our acceptance and celebration.

LET'S UNiTE, NoT FiGHT

I can't help but love this symbolism of the opposites yin and yang co-existing in such complete flow and harmony. It's such a beautiful analogy for the whole of life, as things would seem just so much simpler, and we could all be so much more contented in ourselves, if we could stop competing with, and struggling against, one another and instead just unite, go with the flow and help one another.

To every woman and every man: you are powerful and beautiful as you are. Other people are not our competition, so please let's stand together. While one person can make a difference, together we can rock and change the world. We are at a point in the world where we need different collective messages – powerful ones that encourage mutual support. We need to flood the world with women supporting women and humans supporting humans.

"STEP INTO THE FLOW OF LIFE"

BEAUTIFUL YOU

I'd like to end this chapter by reminding you of just how awesome you are, right now in this moment – no matter what self-doubts you might have, no matter what comments you may, or may not, get from others, whether in either real life or on social media. You are a beautiful balance of incredible universal energies and you deserve to be loved and celebrated.

We are all our own heroes, so let's stop giving our energy away, step into the beautifully flowing river of life and take part in the divine dance before us. This is our world – full of potential for as much love, bravery, beauty and bliss as we are open to receiving. So let's open our hearts and unite in celebrating the wonder of each and every one of us.

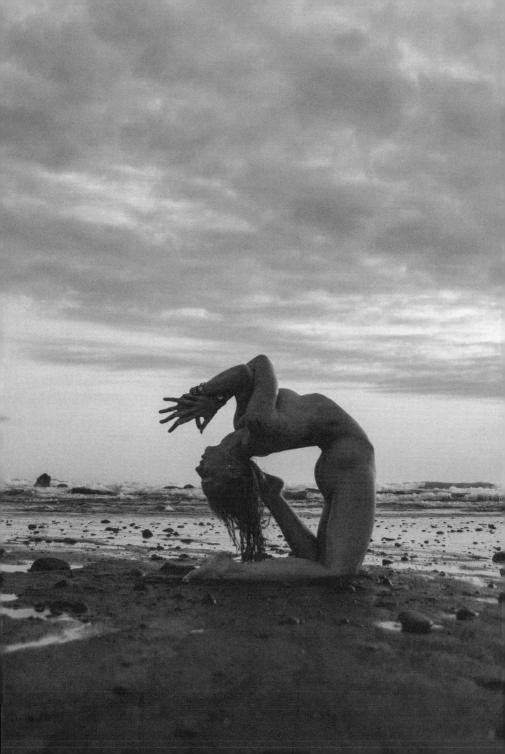

OPENING OUR HEARTS AND LOVING LIFE

CHAPTER 7:
OPENING OUR HEARTS AND LOVING LIFE

We humans can spend our whole lives running from our past hurts, scars and problems, but this means that we ultimately end up running away from our true selves – our freedom, our wholeness and our peace. Our time on this earth is precious, so let's instead choose to open our hearts and celebrate the miracle of being here on this planet while we can.

No one on this earth will ever be able to replace you – you are *epic*, and your warmth, love and kindness are what the world is waiting for. So let this incredible life of yours be about love and happiness. Let it be about falling down and standing back up, about taking chances and having a voice. Let it be about sharing your passion, sensuality and divine sexuality. About being true to yourself, believing in yourself (just like I believe in you) and being a warrior for your beliefs, with the utmost respect and compassion for others.

It's time to open your heart to happiness no matter what life throws at you, shine your light and don't let anything dim it. In this final chapter, we're going to cover several ways to help ourselves do this:

✳ EMBRACING BOTH STRENGTH AND VULNERABILITY
– wouldn't it feel great if we could recognize that each of these
qualities contains a seed of the other, so that there's no need to
beat ourselves up about times when we feel low or doubt ourselves?

**✳ SHARING, SUPPORTING AND LIFTING ONE ANOTHER
UP** – how amazing would it feel to live in a world of mutual trust and
respect, where you knew that everyone around you had your back no
matter what? And where you felt proud to show up for others too?

**✳ CHOOSING A LIFE OF LOVE, BEAUTY, COURAGE AND
UNITY** – isn't it incredible that, ultimately, no matter what we're
given (or not given) in this life, how we experience our time on this
planet is down to us and our own choices? So why not make the most
positive choices we all can to live our best lives from here on in?

If I know one thing, it's that your heart is beautiful, and the Universe
cherishes you. So be brave, be beautiful and bare your soul. We all
love and need each other!

EMBRACING BOTH STRENGTH AND VULNERABILITY

Today's culture often places value on certain qualities and behaviours over others, with a leaning towards all things extrovert, showy and seemingly "strong" and "perfect". As such, many people have never spent time exploring their more vulnerable inner selves, which can make things difficult when we hit hard times. But the truth is that, as the incredible multi-faceted beings that we are, we all have a vulnerable side – and one of the many beauties of life is that we can be both vulnerable in our strength and strong in our vulnerability.

VULNERABILITY AS A STRENGTH

Vulnerability is a funny thing: everyone feels it, yet most people tend to be scared of it. It can come in many forms, and, while it always means being open to hurt and rejection, it's important to remember that it also means being open to much joy, pleasure and learning.

Being vulnerable offers us a chance to be completely honest and authentic, wear our heart on our sleeve, air and heal old wounds, and therefore potentially connect with others in their vulnerabiity, too.

By being strong enough to lay our own selves bare without shame, we help to take away the shame of others and begin to help them be their authentic selves, too. After all, we are all broken and beautiful in our own ways. As such, I personally think vulnerability is one of the greatest often-hidden strengths that we have – and something that the world would benefit from placing more value on.

THE STRENGTH AND VULNERABiLiTY OF AUTHENTiCiTY

As we touched on earlier in the book, at the core of being vulnerable is simply being true to your own inner nature no matter what others might think of this. So if it works for you to do things in a slow and steady way, a crazy and awkward way, or a loud and energetic way, don't let anybody else make you feel that you have to change this and be something you're not just to get their approval. If you enjoy depth, don't *force* yourself to seek breadth or put on a mask of breadth for the sake of others. Instead, celebrate your individuality and never be embarrassed by it. "Baring it all" like this gives you a chance to lean *into* vulnerability, explore it and grow stronger from the experience that unfolds, as tough as it may be at times.

VULNERABiLiTY MEANS HONESTY

Another form of vulnerability is admitting how we've created or received our own scars in life – saying, "I did things that caused me hurt, I'm not proud of it and I've changed", or "I was delivered scars by life, but I'm now taking the responsibility to heal them."

We all hurt ourselves and others tremendously at times, whether intentionally or accidentally. I know I have on many occasions. It's part of being human. But learning to acknowledge and forgive both our own and other people's mistakes with honesty and compassion makes us stronger, not weaker. It's not about the mistakes; it's about how we lean into them and learn to breathe in love again that matters.

INCREDiBLE YOU

Let me remind you once again, dear human, that you are amazing. In your moments of greatest strength, you are amazing. In your moments of greatest vulnerability, you are amazing. So often you might look at what everyone else is doing on the outside and compare yourself from the inside – and this is unfair on yourself. So let me remind you that the brave and beautiful life that you are choosing to live makes a difference. It matters. Every little thing you do matters, especially those moments of utmost vulnerability where you want to whisper, "I quit", but instead you keep on going. That is my definition of strength and being a hero. You are a hero. Every single day. So carry on, superhero! And move through each day – no matter how it goes – remembering that your positive choices will make a difference.

AWESOME BEYOND MEASURE

Remember, life isn't about how much you can lift at the gym or how physically flexible you are. Neither is it about the number of Pinterest projects you complete or the number of Facebook likes you get. Strength isn't rated on a scale of 1 to 10. Instead, it's about giving honestly of your self and loving even when your reserve tank is empty. It's about feeling vulnerable and showing up anyway.

Your family, your friends, your colleagues, that stranger who you smiled at in the street – they all need and value this presence and warmth, this strength and vulnerability. So let's learn to share as openly as we can with each other, and enjoy the ride...

"THIS MOMENT NEEDS YOU"

SHARING, SUPPORTING AND LIFTING ONE ANOTHER UP

With so many obstacles on the road of life, we don't need to create more by getting in our own and one another's way. So one of the things I find most inspiring is when people openly propel each other forward instead of holding each other back.

DARING TO SHARE

I first started blogging when I had deep post-natal depression, both because I felt a need to express myself and I didn't want anyone else to feel as lonely and unhappy as I did. My hope was that when people would see other people, like myself, baring their all with such honesty and vulnerability, that it might make it easier for them to reach out for help and support too.

But sharing ourselves and our stories can be hard. It feels uncomfortable and extremely vulnerable to lay bare our innermost selves in a public way as we are programmed to worry about what others may think and whether or not they will still love and accept us once they know what we perceive to be our vulnerabilities and weaknesses. "Will they still think I'm smart? Beautiful? Funny? A good person? A good mum?" (And so the list goes on.)

WE ARE NOT ALONE

The potential reward, however, is that by both offering support and drawing on the support of others, we can harness the collective energy of our peers to help us feel less alone and therefore less vulnerable –

because, let's face it, it can be rough out there at times, and we're all in this together!

I've talked a lot in this book about the judgement, rejection and abuse that I've been subjected to by people who don't quite "get" what I'm doing as a result of the level to which I've shared myself online. However, I also want to acknowledge just how immeasurably harder I know my journey through my challenges would have been without the incredible support of the rest of my amazing online community who have been there to lift and inspire me along the way.

So I want to thank you from the bottom of my heart. Thank you for helping to lift me when I most needed it and for allowing me to try to do the same for you. That kind of love is a humbling gift to receive.

BE THE CHANGE WE WANT TO SEE

So often the news is filled with stories of people judging and hurting one another instead of loving and supporting one another. So let's continue to be the change we want to see – part of the wider movement to create a kinder, more sustainable world that is based on more love, beauty, courage and unity (over hatred, ugliness, fear and separation).

I've written a letter on the page overleaf that I hope will help you feel at least a little less alone and a little more supported if ever you need a boost from a friend.

Please come back to this any time it might help. Also feel free to copy it and pass it forward to anyone you know who may benefit from its message of love and support. It is a letter for anyone who has had a rough day, week, year or more; who seems to be under a cloud at the moment; who feels invisible and trodden on; who feels tired and worn down by life; or who might have lost their faith and feel like giving up...

<u>Dear friend</u>

I know you may not feel it right now,
but you are awesome, beautiful and amazing.

I see all that you are, so please know that
your energy, stamina, endurance, dedication,
commitment, sense of purpose and, above all,
sacrifice, do not go unnoticed.

I am proud of you. If I was living your life,
I wouldn't know how to do it as marvellously
as you. You make this world more beautiful,
you have so much potential and so many
wonderful things still left to do.

Better things are coming your way, so hang in
there. By opening our hearts and
supporting each other, together, we can make
the rest of our lives the best of our lives.

I know you've got this!
Love & blessings,
Rhy

CHOOSING A LIFE OF LOVE, BEAUTY, COURAGE AND UNITY

We don't need to chase extraordinary moments to find happiness. All the happiness we need is right here in front of us; we just need to choose to open our hearts and live our own truths with acceptance and gratitude to discover a life of love, beauty, courage and unity that exceeds our wildest dreams.

BELIEVING IN THE MAGIC AND LOOKING FOR THE LOVE

Life can be full of magic and love, but only if we take a leap of faith and make a conscious decision to believe in magic in the first place. Only then can we start to find "magical" loving solutions to problems. Only then can we accept that just because we sometimes can't *find* a definitive answer, it doesn't mean that there's no answer at all.

Today, let's remove any jaded, sceptical spectacles that we've been inadvertently wearing and instead try watching the world with fresh, sparkling, heart-led eyes that will find where the love is.

EMBRACING THE BEAUTIFUL MESSINESS OF IT ALL

People sometimes ask me, "How do you do it all?" The answer is simple: I don't! Nobody does. Whenever you see someone succeeding in one area of their life, they are almost certainly struggling, even if only minorly, in another. If I am killing it in my yoga practice, then I am probably behind in my day-to-day parenting. And if I am being an awesome mama, I am probably being challenged somewhere else in my hobbies and life.

"BE BRAVE. BE BEAUTIFUL. LET THE WORLD SEE YOU"

We can't do it *all*; we can just do our best, one loving breath at a time. And this is enough. This is a life of beauty.

For me these days, beauty is in the eyes, the smile and the heart – in the way someone shows their love. It is not a look, a set of curves, a pose or a way of walking, but in how brightly we allow ourselves, and others, to shine! Beauty is being kind, compassionate and loving to both ourselves and others. It is knowing that we are enough! And it is the choice to make other souls soar and therefore make all of our lives more exciting and wonderful.

HAVING THE COURAGE TO BE SEEN

Let's all be brave, worthy and amazing. Every single time we get the chance, let's stand up in front of people – even if we are, by nature, an introvert. Let them see us. Let's speak and be heard. Let's persevere despite the dry mouth and the fast heartbeat. Let's take it all in and breathe this rare air. That way, we can feel alive and be ourselves. You are truly, finally, always yourself. And that's enough.

THE POWER OF GRATITUDE

As mentioned earlier in the book (page 53), our sense of love, beauty and courage can all be enhanced if we choose to live a life of conscious gratitude. Wherever we are, and whoever we are with, with practice, we can nearly always find something that makes our hearts sing and our souls thankful. So let's never forget to thank the people who make us feel on top of the world and to acknowledge all the moments, activities and other things that make life feel truly stunning. These are what will keep our self-belief strong, our heads in the stars, and our hearts and souls soaring even amidst the storms of life.

Flick over two pages and you will find an exercise to help you develop an "attitude of gratitude" that will help you to live in this optimal way, truly loving life, whatever it brings you.

THE UNITY OF ALL THINGS

When we actively choose the combination of all the positive qualities that we have explored in this book, we are choosing to truly open up to life, be ourselves, connect with others in a sense of unity – and live our best lives.

WALKING YOUR OWN PATH

I take my hat off to all you epic souls who are out there being your authentic selves, chasing your dreams, owning your failures, trying new things, getting out of your comfort zones, and taking responsibility for being the change you wish to see in the world while celebrating others for doing the same.

You are the people who make the difference. For everything that now exists was once considered impossible, yet here it is. So keep the faith in your vision, whatever it may be.

THE JOURNEY SO FAR

You have already come so far. And, if you're anything like me, I know that you are likely to be juggling a lot – determined to make your time count, to be as efficient and organized as you can, to thoughtfully and purposefully arrange your priorities; and to live in a way that will not only give you the best shot at personal happiness, but that you also believe will make the world a better place, in whatever small a measure.

By choosing to pick up this book and go on this journey of being "brave, beautiful and baring it all" with me, you are making a difference. So I want you to know that you are admired for this – for all that you manage and all that you give. You may well crave more time – to spend with those you love, to exercise more, to rest more... I know your time is precious. But the world needs you, beautiful soul, and I feel so grateful to have connected with you in these pages.

BE BRAVE, BE BEAUTIFUL AND BARE IT ALL

Please never believe anyone who tells you that you're not enough. If ever you feel like you're struggling, remember that somewhere in this world there is a girl called Rhyanna (that's me!) – and that this girl supports you and loves you just as you are, in all your bravery, in all your beauty and even when you "bare it all" – in fact, *especially* when you "bare it all"!

So thank you for having embarked on the journey through this book with me. Thank you for being your authentic amazing self. Thank you for opening your heart to my thoughts, insights and messages. I hope that you have found some element of comfort, reassurance and food for thought in the words that will help you to continue on your own journey of love, light, bravery, beauty and inspiration.

DEVELOPING AN ATTITUDE OF GRATITUDE

If practised regularly, the exercise below can really start to shift your mindset to focusing on what you're already lucky enough to *have* and *be* in life rather than what you don't have or what you'd like to be more of.

1. When you wake up in the morning, take a moment to sit in silence, breathe deeply and settle into your self.

2. Once you're in a nice calm rhythm of breathing, start to feel into and acknowledge the many beautiful things you have in life right now, and inhale with a sense of deep gratitude for each one of these things that comes to mind.

3. Without judgement, visualize yourself exhaling any negativity that challenges each positive thought.

4. Continue this for as long as feels comfortable, breathing in with love while focusing on what is wonderful, and letting go of any fear or restrictions as you breathe out.

5. When you are ready, bow your head slightly in a final small nod of gratitude, staying here for a few moments to acknowledge your place in the incredible wider world.

6. Then, when you're ready, head out to embrace whatever the day has in store for you, knowing that you *have* and *are* everything you need within you, all the while still recognizing, of course, that there is always potential for further change and growth.

Using this exercise each morning to develop an "attitude of gratitude" has immense power to transform the way you experience each day – so that you see and accept events that unfold with more love, compassion, joy and positivity.

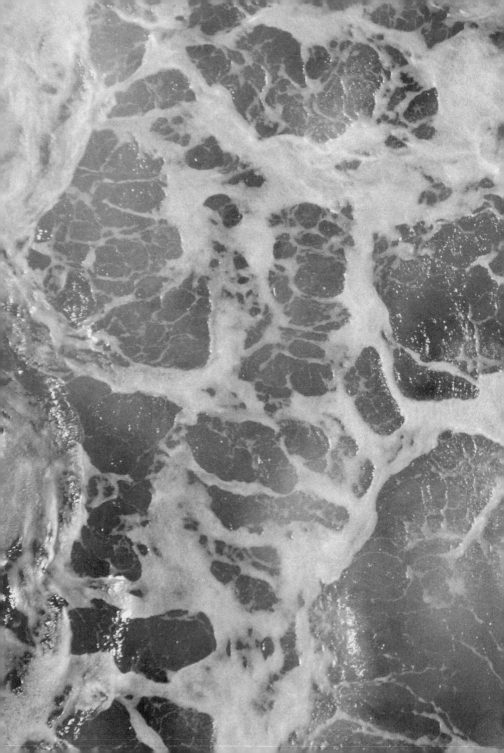

AFTERWORD

I'd like to add a final little extra note just to remind you that, despite the words of insight that I've offered you in the pages of this book, I'm still very much finding my own perfectly imperfect way – alongside you – on the brave and beautiful journey of life.

Like everyone, I'm constantly being faced with new challenges. And I still find it hard to confront the ways in which some of my old traumas raise their ugly heads within me at times. So, for example, it still feels tough some days to focus on all the amazing positive interactions that I'm lucky enough to have and not to feel hurt, upset or broken by criticisms and rejections. But I'm happy to say that, on the whole, I'm now able to much more quickly get out of my head and into a loving heart space in which I can enjoy a wider, more beautiful view of the world – with a sense of awe, wonder and gratitude.

And while I'm sometimes afraid to share my journey, as I know it won't resonate with everyone, I would like to iterate once again just how incredibly grateful I feel for the support of each and every one of you – the community of open hearts that has united around my sharing. It gives me hope that this world is full of shining people whose light will help my daughter, Laine, find her way on her own path.

If you listen closely to the sound you hear if you ever feel that you have shattered, know that it is the music from the birth of your wings, rippling through your spine. This is your chance to take flight.

All my love and blessings,
Rhy

APPENDIX: BREATHE INTO YOUR BRAVERY AND BEAUTY

As we've explored throughout this book, being brave doesn't mean we have to jump out of planes or fight lions! It simply means being open enough to really get to know and love ourselves, stripped of societal pressures and expectations. And as for being beautiful, we're all beautiful in our own ways, so it's just about accepting and embracing this.

However, these things are easier said than done, so now that we've journeyed together through a range of approaches that I hope will help you on this path, I'd like to return to the power of the breath which we touched on in the introduction.

On the pages that follow you will find a range of simple breathing meditations – one relating to each of the chapters in the book – to help you really relax into each way of being. But first, a few breath meditation tips to get you started:

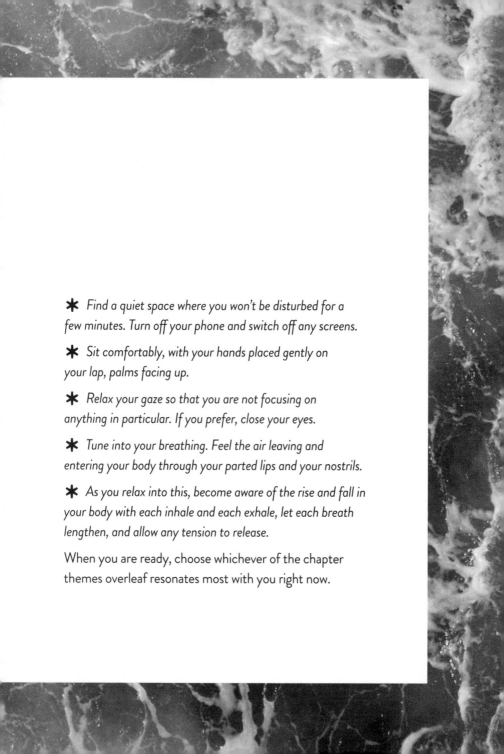

✱ *Find a quiet space where you won't be disturbed for a few minutes. Turn off your phone and switch off any screens.*

✱ *Sit comfortably, with your hands placed gently on your lap, palms facing up.*

✱ *Relax your gaze so that you are not focusing on anything in particular. If you prefer, close your eyes.*

✱ *Tune into your breathing. Feel the air leaving and entering your body through your parted lips and your nostrils.*

✱ *As you relax into this, become aware of the rise and fall in your body with each inhale and each exhale, let each breath lengthen, and allow any tension to release.*

When you are ready, choose whichever of the chapter themes overleaf resonates most with you right now.

1. LAYING OUR AUTHENTIC SELVES BARE

As you sit and breathe, remember that the art of discovering, and being willing to share, your authentic self begins with accepting and loving yourself. You might have been conditioned to judge yourself harshly from a young age. You might have been taught to starve your soul and feed your ego. Now it's time to feed your soul again – with love. So, with each inhale, picture yourself breathing in love – pure, unconditional love, whatever that looks like for you. And, with each exhale, breathe out any obstacles that stand in its way.

2. SEEING THE PERFECTION IN IMPERFECTION

As you sit and breathe, consider how much you look to others to mirror back love and affection into your life, rather than recognizing the imperfect perfection of your own incredible reflection. With each inhale, say silently to yourself, "I am enough, I am worthy, I am perfect as I am." And with each exhale, say thank you but farewell to the voice of the negative inner critic inside your head.

3. CHOOSING COMPASSION OVER STORIES IN OUR HEAD

As you sit and breathe, ask yourself: What if I accepted myself and others fully, with love and kindness, rather than judging and resenting due to limiting thoughts in my own head? With each inhale, picture yourself breathing in love and forgiveness. And with each exhale, let go of anything that brings you disappointment, shame, anger or regret.

4. FREEING OUR INNER CHILD

As you sit and breathe, consider what emotional walls you may have built around yourself from your life experiences to date. Picture yourself dismantling these brick by brick to leave yourself in the open space in which you were born. With each inhale, breathe in a sense of the freedom and endless possibilities that lie before you – and see yourself embracing this with a sense of curiosity and playfulness. And with each exhale, breathe out any remaining sense of being trapped by fear and conditioning.

5. REALIZING DARKNESS ALLOWS OUR LIGHT TO SHINE

As you sit and breathe, take time to acknowledge the fact that both day and night, light and darkness, have their place in this world. Without one, the value of the other would be diminished. With each inhale, breathe in a sense of complete acceptance of all that you are, both your light *and* your shadow sides. And with each exhale, allow any fear of, or resistance to, the darker aspects of yourself to fade away.

6. EMBRACING OUR INNATE SENSUALITY

As you sit and breathe, acknowledge your incredible body as the temple that it is, allowing you to live, feel and physically connect with this wonderful world and the people in it. With each inhale, breathe in a sense of gratitude at everything you get to enjoy each day through the wonder of your senses. And with each exhale, breathe out any sense of resistance you may have to embracing the full range of pleasure that embracing your innate sensuality can bring to your life.

7. OPENING OUR HEARTS AND LOVING LIFE

As you sit and breathe, immerse yourself in the knowledge that we are all, ultimately, one – and that our differences are there to connect us, not separate us. When we open our hearts and love one another as one big family, we get to see the magic that lies in others as well as ourselves. With each inhale, feel a sense of your heart opening to the wonder of the world. And with each exhale, simply relax into this feeling of love and expansiveness.

Please feel free to do these breathing meditations – and/or reread the associated chapters – any time you feel you could do with a little help getting out of your own head and more into your body and heart.

I hope they'll encourage you to find the inspiration within your own beautiful heart and soul to live a life that you truly love – full of authenticity, compassion, connection and unity; bravery, beauty and baring it all.

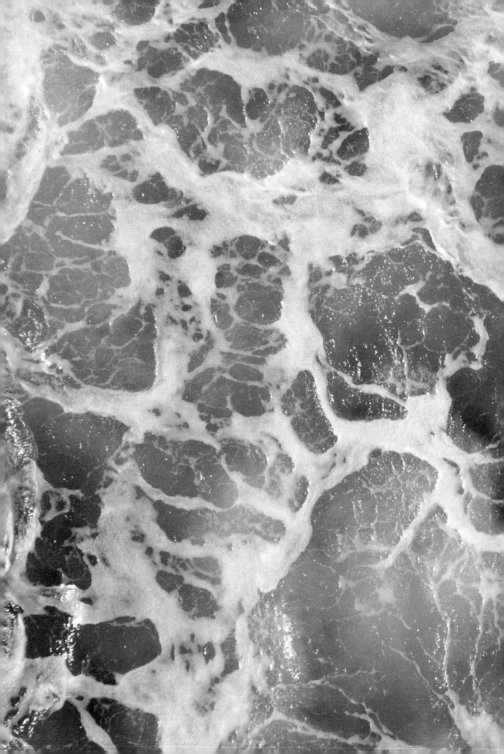

FURTHER INSPIRATION

I have read many books that have inspired me to keep living as bravely and as beautifully as possible, with both an open heart and an open mind. Below is a selection of some of my most recent reads in the hope that you might enjoy, and benefit from, them as much as I did...

Boehm, Michaela, *The Wild Woman's Way*, 2018

Brown, Brené, *The Gifts of Imperfection*, 2018

Collins, Mel, *The Handbook for Highly Sensitive People*, 2019

Finn, Eoin, *Blissology Teacher Training Manual*.

Frankl, Viktor E. *Man's Search for Meaning*, Gift Edition, 2014

Gill, Nikita, *Your Soul is a River*, 2018

Kalanithti, Paul, *When Breath Becomes Air*, 2017

Lee, Becca, *Becoming Beautiful*, 2018

Markul, Tanya, *The She Book*, 2019

McGill, Bryant. *Simple Reminders: Inspiration for Living Your Best Life*, 2015

Obama, Michelle, *Becoming*, 2018

Perel, Esther, *Mating in Captivity: Unlocking Erotic Intelligence*, 2007

Perel, Esther, *The State of Affairs: Rethinking Infidelity*, 2017

Pueblo, Yung, *Inward*, 2017

Purdy, Amy, *On My Own Two Feet*, 2015

Rhimes, Shonda, *Year of Yes*, 2016

Robinson, Janne, *This is for the Women Who Don't Give a Fuck*, 2019

Rousey, Ronda, *My Fight Your Fight*, 2016

Sadhguru, *Inner Engineering: A Yogi's Guide to Joy*, 2016

Sparacino, Bianca, *The Strength in Our Scars*, 2018

Stabile, Scott, *Big Love: The Power of Living with a Wide-Open Heart*, 2017

West, Brianna, *101 Essays that will Change the way You Think*, 2018

ACKNOWLEDGEMENTS

With thanks first to my beautiful daughter, Laine. I hope you know how awesome you are. I hope as you grow you will always remember your deepest dreams and the things that make your soul laugh out loud. Never forget the reasons why you made the choices you have and, most importantly, always walk with your head high, shoulders low and a smile on your dial because you are so magnificent. You make me a better human. You show me happiness is the way, not a goal. You remind me every day that the small things are the big things and love is all we need. My life is rich not in paper but in what matters because of you. I am blessed beyond words – and every day you remind me of this. Namaste, my beautiful angel, you are the greatest gift and miracle life has ever given me!

Thank you, too, to my mum, dad and brother for always shining light into my life, reminding me that I am worthy even if it feels like the world is saying otherwise. Thank you, Martin, my partner in crime, for tolerating my idiosyncracies and crazy Tassie Devil ways. You might not know this, but you helped me find my true self and my happiness. And thanks also to the Rainbachers – your love is a special gift, generously given, happily received and deeply appreciated.

Without the people around me in my life and the people I've connected with online, this book would never have come to light. So, to every person who has touched my life, I want to thank you from the bottom of my heart, because I am the sum total of my experiences with each one of you. Good or bad, I am where I am today because of you and my family and friends standing by me. I am always most astounded, moved and transported by the warmth and kindness of a loving person. Always.

Most heartfelt thanks also to my amazing editors Kelly and Sue for all your awesomeness – and to Kelly for guiding me gently through the whole process of making this book. I read my text full of emotion and joy at your ability to help my voice come across in a harmonious way. Thank you for helping me fulfill my passion in life – to leave footprints in the sand for a kinder world for my beautiful daughter. You are not only epic people but you are making Laine's future more full of love and light, and for this I am forever grateful.

A big thank you also to everyone else at Watkins, from Etan for having made initial contact with me and the design team for creating both the beautiful cover and interior layouts, to the production, sales, marketing and publicity departments for all their invaluable contributions. You are all magic makers.

And finally an enormous thank you to Olivia, the beautiful soul and amazing photographer I met in Bali, whose black-and-white images really help add another whole beautiful and vital dimension to the book. I am immensely grateful for your creativity and artistry.

Thank you all from the bottom of my open heart! May this book that we have created together encourage more hearts to open even just a little further in pursuit of the freedom, happiness and fulfilment that we're all looking for.

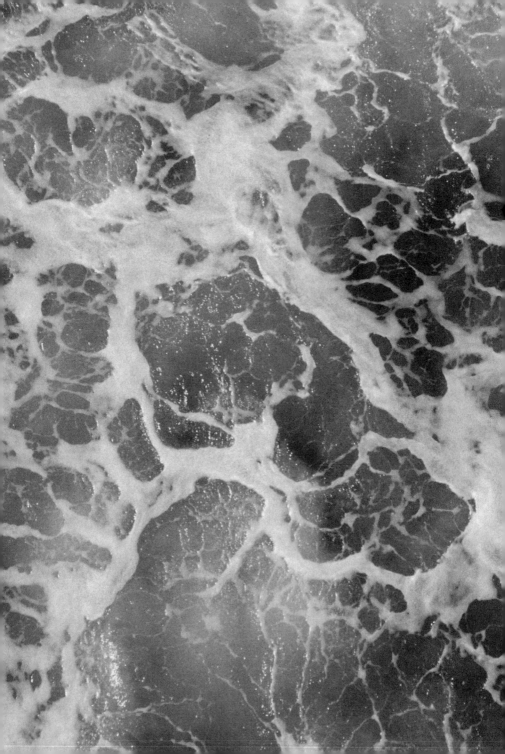

ABOUT THE AUTHOR

Rhyanna Watson is a fitness trainer, yoga teacher, wellness consultant, mum, Instagrammer and YouTuber, who has had a love of all things health- and fitness-related from a young age, and who is humbled and astounded by the extensive community of like-minded souls and open hearts who have come together to exchange ideas, support and inspire one another on her online platform.

She has both played water polo and swam for Tasmania, competed in track at the Pan-Pacific Games and been a fitness director on cruise ships, and she now offers a range of online wellness programmes.

She has come out the other side of personal traumas, including sexual assault, the loss of her first baby, post-natal depression and a suicide attempt, both stronger and happier.

Originally from Tasmania but now based in Switzerland, she loves engaging with her online community at Open Hearts Can Unite, challenging mainstream perceptions of female fitness and sensuality, and helping her followers to be brave enough to live in ways that they previously only dreamt of – fit, open, vibrant, contented, true to themselves and free.

If you would like to connect further with Rhyanna, her training and online community, you can do so via:
www.rhyannawatson.com
Instagram: @openheartscanunite
or her YouTube Channel: Open Hearts Can Unite

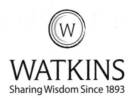

WATKINS

Sharing Wisdom Since 1893

The story of Watkins began in 1893, when scholar of esotericism John Watkins founded our bookshop, inspired by the lament of his friend and teacher Madame Blavatsky that there was nowhere in London to buy books on mysticism, occultism or metaphysics. That moment marked the birth of Watkins, soon to become the publisher of many of the leading lights of spiritual literature, including Carl Jung, Rudolf Steiner, Alice Bailey and Chögyam Trungpa.

Today, the passion at Watkins Publishing for vigorous questioning is still resolute. Our stimulating and groundbreaking list ranges from ancient traditions and complementary medicine to the latest ideas about personal development, holistic wellbeing and consciousness exploration. We remain at the cutting edge, committed to publishing books that change lives.

DISCOVER MORE AT:

www.watkinspublishing.com

Read our blog   Watch and listen to   Sign up to
our authors in action   our mailing list

We celebrate conscious, passionate, wise and happy living.
Be part of that community by visiting

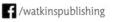 /watkinspublishing   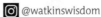 @watkinswisdom
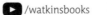 /watkinsbooks   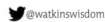 @watkinswisdom